UNIVERSAL HEALER

BOOK 2
TYPE II DIABETES

Dr Larry Lytle

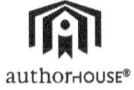

authorHOUSE®

AuthorHouse™
1663 Liberty Drive
Bloomington, IN 47403
www.authorhouse.com
Phone: 1-800-839-8640

First published by AuthorHouse   10/14/2011

ISBN: 978-1-4670-5430-0 (sc)
ISBN: 978-1-4670-7092-8 (e)

Library of Congress Control Number: 2011917785

Printed in the United States of America

Health is a state of complete physical,
mental and social well-being, and not
merely the absence of disease or infirmity.

World Health Organization
1948

Author's Notes

First they ignore you,
then they laugh at you,
then they fight you,
then you win.

Mahatma Gandhi

It is with great pleasure that I present *Universal Healer: Book 2 Type II Diabetes*, on the heels of two successes: *Universal Healer: Book 1 Osteoarthritis,* and FDA approval of the QLaser for the treatment of osteoarthritis of the hand (see letter that follows). The latter, for me, is a triumph in my quest to help heal the world more safely. This is just the beginning. I look forward to having a QLaser in every home by the year 2035, and then the whole body will be healed with energy.

Department of Health & Human Services
Public Health Service
Food & Drug Administration
9200 Corporate Boulevard
Rockville, MD 20850

Jan 30 2009

2035, Inc.
c/o Regulatory Insight Incorporated
Mr. Kevin Walls
13 Red Fox Lane
Littleton, Colorado 80127

Re: K080513
Trade/Device Name: QLaser System
Regulation Number: 21 CFR 890.5500
Regulation Name: Infrared lamp
Regulatory Class: II
Product Code: NHN
Dated: January 9, 2009
Received: January 12, 2009

Dear Mr. Walls:

We have reviewed your Section 510(k) premarket notification of intent to market the device referenced above and have determined the device is substantially equivalent (for the indications for use stated in the enclosure) to legally marketed predicate devices marketed in interstate commerce prior to May 28, 1976, the enactment date of the Medical Device Amendments, or to devices that have been reclassified in accordance with the provisions of the Federal Food, Drug, and Cosmetic Act (Act) that do not require approval of a premarket approval application (PMA). You may, therefore, market the device, subject to the general controls provisions of the Act. The general controls provisions of the Act include requirements for annual registration, listing of devices, good manufacturing practice, labeling, and prohibitions against misbranding and adulteration.

If your device is classified (see above) into either class II (Special Controls) or class III (PMA), it may be subject to such additional controls. Existing major regulations affecting your device can be found in the Code of

Federal Regulations, Title 21, Parts 800 to 898. In addition, FDA may publish further announcements concerning your device in the <u>Federal Register.</u>

Please be advised that FDA's issuance of a substantial equivalence determination does not mean that FDA has made a determination that your device complies with other requirements of the Act or any Federal statutes and regulations administered by other Federal agencies. You must comply with all the Act's requirements, including, but not limited to: registration and listing (21 CFR Part 807); labeling (21 CFR Part 801); good manufacturing practice requirements as set forth in the quality systems (QS) regulation (21 CFR Part 820); and if applicable, the electronic product radiation control provisions (Sections 531-542 of the Act); 21 CFR 1000-1050.

This letter will allow you to begin marketing your device as described in your Section 510(k) premarket notification. The FDA finding of substantial equivalence of your device to a legally marketed predicate device results in a classification for your device and thus, permits your device to proceed to market.

If you desire specific advice for your device on our labeling regulation (21 CFR Part 801), please contact the Center for Devices and Radiological Health's (CDRH's) Office of Compliance...

Indications for Use
Device Name: QLaser System

Indications for use: The QLaser System is indicated for providing temporary relief of pain associated with osteoarthritis of the hand, which has been diagnosed by a physician or other licensed medical professional.

Sincerely yours,
Mark N. Melkerson
Director
Division of General, Restorative
And Neurological Devices
Office of Device Evaluation
Center for Devices and Radiological Health

INTRODUCTION

He who has health has hope; and
he who has hope has everything.

Arabic proverb

Diabetes, including Type I and Type II, has been around for many years, but newly diagnosed cases in the past decade went through the roof, at approximately a 90 percent rate increase over the previous decade, a problem of epidemic proportions. The culprits: obesity and sedentary lifestyles, according to U. S. health officials. Apparently, they see no end to the diabetes epidemic any time soon.

Here are some startling facts about diabetes:

- Eight percent of the U.S. population (23.6 million children and adults) has one form or another of diabetes, according to the American Diabetes Association. From 2005-2007 the prevalence of diabetes cases increased 13.5 percent.

- The leading cause of diabetes-related deaths is heart disease.

- Diabetics face a heightened risk of developing heart disease, stroke, kidney damage, and blindness.

- Approximately 73 percent of diabetic adults also have been diagnosed with high blood pressure and/or is dependent on prescription medications to control hypertension.

- For adult diabetics between the ages of 20 and 74, diabetes is the leading cause of new cases of blindness.

- Especially for Type II diabetics, proper diet and nutrition can play an important role in controlling diabetes.

- Approximately 60 percent to 70 percent of diabetics suffer from mild to severe forms of nerve system damage.

- More than 60 percent of limb amputations (not caused by trauma) occur in diabetics.

- As of 2002, almost 45,000 diabetics began treatment for end-stage renal failure.

- Also, approximately 154,000 people were living on chronic kidney dialysis or with a kidney transplant.

- No longer a disease of the elderly, diabetes has invaded the lives of younger people, even children, at an alarming rate; in fact, according to the International Diabetes Foundation, Type II diabetes in children is becoming a global public health issue.

As you can see, diabetes—whether Type I or Type II—is a serious medical condition that cannot go untreated. Type II diabetes, the most common form, is closely linked to obesity. The alarming spike in Type II diabetes in recent years is in direct correlation to the rise in obesity, and the concern now is that there has been a 90 percent to 95 percent increase of new Type II cases in juveniles, over Type I.

The rise in Type II diabetes cases appears to be regionally skewed; the highest number of new cases comes from the southern states: Alabama, Florida, Georgia, Kentucky, Louisiana, South Carolina, Tennessee, Texas, and West Virginia. The greatest number of new cases came from West Virginia (12.7 per 1,000 people). High fat, high sugar diets in people who live in the southern states should be noted, as there is a considerably higher percentage of obesity in those populations; this is important since obesity and Type II diabetes are linked. It goes without saying that efforts to prevent Type II diabetes should be concentrated in these states. The people in Minnesota might serve as an example; that state reported the lowest number of new cases (only 5 per 1,000).

An important fact arose in the report issued in October 2008: while doctors have been using newer and more expensive drugs to treat diabetes, there is little long-term evidence that they work better than older, less expensive medications, as you will see in Chapter 2. This fact opens the door for alternative treatments, such as low level laser treatment, the focus of this book.

Now the good news: It is no secret that Type II diabetes especially starts when insulin cannot get into the cells to make cellular energy called ATP. From that point on, bad things happen. Theories abound as to why trillions of cells do not allow insulin to enter them, <u>but today there is hope</u>. This hope rests on an entirely different philosophy: no drugs, no blaming obesity, lack of exercise or heredity, and no need for kidney failure, amputation or surgery.

The right kind and combination of laser light restores electrons and activates production of nitric oxide, which transports insulin across cell membranes and enhances production of ATP. Some studies show that laser light not only activates production of ATP, but also cures diabetes and heals the pancreas, heart, kidney and other organs.

Energy manifested by the right combination of laser light may be the biggest breakthrough in health, ever. This safe, economical, easy-to-apply self-therapy will change humankind. The pharmaceutical industry and organized medicine will be slow to accept such simple and harmless self-treatment. It is up to you to "take charge" and awaken the doctor within.

Did you know?

- By the year 2025, more than 380 million people worldwide will have been diagnosed with diabetes.

- The United States, with 23.4 million diabetics, ranks third among all nations, trailing India (first) and China (second).

- Each year, another 7 million people will be diagnosed with diabetes.

- Every 10 seconds, two people develop diabetes.

CONTENTS

Chapter 1

What is Type II Diabetes?

A wise man should consider
that health is the greatest
of human blessings, and learn
how by his own thought to
derive benefit from his illnesses.

Hippocrates
460-377 BC

There are three forms of diabetes. Type I diabetes, the least common condition, is characterized by little or no production of insulin by the pancreas. It is generally thought that a person with Type I diabetes needs to take insulin injections for life, however a 2010 study in Russia shows that using a combination of low level laser diodes reduces blood sugar levels of Type I diabetes and Type II diabetes.

Type II diabetes or Diabetes Mellitus, which was once referred to as or adult-onset or non-insulin-dependent diabetes, is a chronic condition that affects the body's metabolism of sugar (glucose), which is our primary source of fuel. This disease can be debilitating and is sometimes fatal.

The third type of diabetes develops during pregnancy and usually goes away after childbirth; this type is known as gestational diabetes.

CAUSES

Our bodies are comprised of myriad cells that make up our muscles and other tissues. Glucose derived from the food we eat and from our liver, is the main energy source of these cells. Digestion enables sugar to become absorbed into the bloodstream and then into the cells with the help of insulin.

The pancreas, a gland located behind the stomach, secretes insulin into the bloodstream. As this vital hormone circulates, it serves as a catalyst, allowing sugar to enter the cells. Insulin lowers the amount of sugar in the bloodstream. (We have already mentioned problems that arise when excessive sugar remains in the blood). As the blood sugar level drops, the pancreas cuts back its secretion of insulin.

Another vital organ is the liver, which stores glucose for those times when your insulin level drops—such as when you have not eaten in awhile. That is when the liver opens the gate and releases stored glucose to keep your glucose level within a normal range.

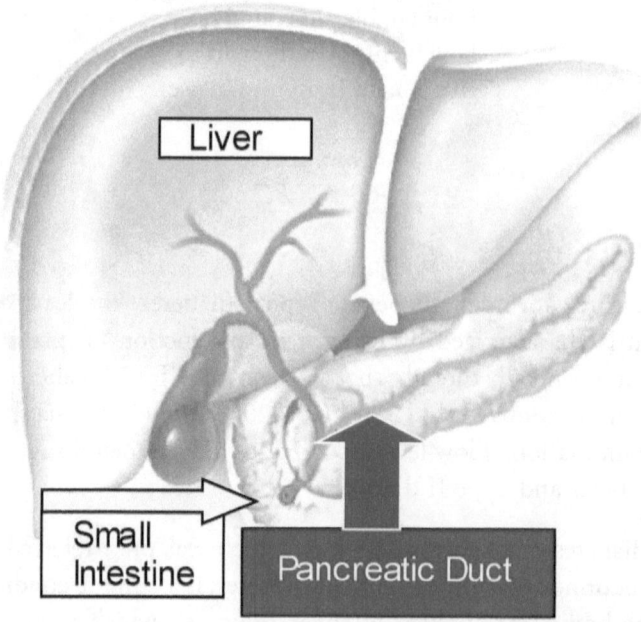

©2009 WebMD, LLC

For Type II diabetic people, this whole process doesn't work right. Sugar is blocked from moving into their cells; it builds up in their bloodstream;

and then the pancreas cannot manufacture enough insulin or their cells become resistant to the action of insulin. We really don't know exactly why this happens, but it seems that excess fat—especially abdominal fat—and inactivity are important factors to help explain it.

TYPE II DIABETES – STEP BY STEP

Here is what happens in the Type II diabetic:

1. The digestive process changes food into glucose.

2. From there, the glucose enters the bloodstream.

3. The pancreas produces insulin.

4. Insulin enters the bloodstream.

5. Cells become insulin-resistant; insulin cannot enter the cell.

6. Eventually the pancreas gradually stops producing insulin and without enough insulin, the glucose cannot get into the body's cells, and it builds up in the blood vessels.

We do know that either inadequate production of insulin or insulin-resistance prevents glucose from entering the body's cells, resulting in build-up of glucose in the blood, causing improper functioning of the cells, among other problems, such as dehydration, diabetic coma, and damage to many of the body's vital organs.

Dehydration occurs when the build-up of sugar triggers increased urination. When losing excess glucose through urine, the body also loses a large amount of water. Severe dehydration happens when the Type II diabetic cannot drink enough fluids to replenish the loss. This can lead to diabetic coma, a life-threatening medical emergency rendering the person unconscious due to acute complications, such as a severe high glucose level (hyperglycemia) in the blood and not enough glucose in the cells (hypoglycemia). It is estimated that 2 to 15 percent of diabetics will have at least one episode of diabetic coma.

Left untreated or improperly treated, the presence of high glucose levels in the blood can result in damage to nerves, small blood vessels of the eyes, kidneys, and heart, and predispose the person to hardening of the large arteries that can cause heart attacks and strokes.

RISK FACTORS

Just about anyone is at risk of developing Type II diabetes, but certain risk factors, if present in any combination, heighten the risk. The primary risk factors are:

- Obesity or being overweight—an excessive amount of fatty tissue makes your cells more resistant to insulin, thereby heightening the risk of Type II diabetes

- Sedentary lifestyle—makes it harder to control your weight, use up glucose as energy, and make your cells more sensitive to insulin

- A history of gestational diabetes—for women who had gestational diabetes when they were pregnant or if they delivered a baby weighing nine pounds or more

- Genetics—having family members (parents or siblings) who have Type II diabetes

- Race (African Americans, Hispanics, Native Americans, and Asian Americans)

- Metabolic syndrome, a cluster of problems, such as high cholesterol, high triglycerides, low good HDL cholesterol, high bad LDL cholesterol, and high blood pressure

- Aging, which makes the body less tolerant of sugars, especially after the age of forty-five, due in part to less exercise, loss of muscle mass, and weight gain; the exception is in the current alarming increase of Type II diabetes among children, adolescents, and younger adults

- Pre-diabetes, a higher than normal blood sugar level, but not in the range of Type II diabetes; if untreated, pre-diabetes can progress to Type II diabetes. The CDC estimates that seventy-nine million Americans are pre-diabetic.

PREVENTION & MANAGEMENT OF BLOOD SUGAR

At this time, orthodox western medicine does not believe there is a cure for Type II diabetes, but there are many ways that a person can prevent the condition altogether or manage their blood sugar:

- Eating healthy foods

- Making physical exercise a daily routine

- Maintaining a healthy weight

- Taking diabetes medications

- Undergoing insulin therapy

- Utilizing QLaser System therapy on a regular basis

Although progression among those with pre-diabetes is not inevitable, studies indicate that pre-diabetics who lose weight and increase physical activity can prevent or at least delay the onset of diabetes and even return their blood glucose levels to normal. In the Diabetes Prevention Program, a large prevention study of high-risk people for diabetes, lifestyle intervention and behavior modification reduced the development of diabetes by 58 percent over three years; even greater in people sixty years and older, the rate was 71 percent.

Another significant incentive for interventions to prevent or delay Type II diabetes in pre-diabetic individuals is the cost-effectiveness; research has shown that behavior modification is more cost-effective than treatment medications. Translation: It costs less to maintain good health and lower the risk of Type II diabetes than it costs to treat it once it is diagnosed. You will learn that the QLaser System is an economical way to self-treat diabetes.

Moreover, failure to control Type II diabetes can result in any number of serious or life-threatening problems, including:

- Retinopathy, an extension of abnormalities and other eye problems in people with Type II diabetes; progression of this problem can be prevented by controlling sugar, blood pressure, and cholesterol.

- Kidney damage, a risk that increases over time (the longer a person has Type II diabetes, the greater the risk of this problem, which, in its most advanced state, can bring about kidney failure and heart disease.

- Poor blood circulation and nerve damage, which can lead to increased infections and risk of ulcers, heightening the risk of amputation. Nerve damage can also increase risk of digestive problems – nausea, vomiting, and diarrhea.

SYMPTOMS

While many unsuspecting people are diagnosed with diabetes during an apparently unrelated medical crisis, others should be aware of any number of symptoms, which vary from individual to individual, and which are unexplained (not attributed to another factor or factors):

- Increased thirst

- Increased hunger, especially after eating

- Dry mouth

- Weight loss

- Nausea and occasional vomiting

- Frequent urination

- Fatigue (feeling weak and tired)

- Blurred vision

- Numbness or tingling of hands and feet

- Frequent infections of the skin, urinary tract or vagina

- Slow healing of sores, minor cuts, or frequent infections

Increased thirst and frequent urination result, as the build-up of excess sugar in the blood causes fluid to be pulled from the body's tissues, leaving the person thirsty. Typically, one's thirst calls for more fluids, and therefore more urination.

Extreme hunger is triggered when the body's muscles and organs become depleted of energy, due to insulin resistance or not enough insulin to allow sugar to enter the cell, and the cell does not produce enough energy (ATP). When this problem persists even after a person has eaten, it could indicate the presence of Type II diabetes.

Even though a person eats more to satisfy constant hunger, he or she may lose weight, which is due to shrinkage of muscle tissues and fat stores that have insufficient energy or ATP. If the body's cells do not have sufficient glucose (sugar) to make cellular ATP (energy), the person can become tired and irritable.

Blurred vision results when the blood sugar level is too high, causing fluid to be pulled from the body's tissues, including the eye lenses. Another symptom, perhaps more alarming, is the change in how cuts and sores heal or how often the person experiences infections. Type II diabetes affects the body's ability to heal and fight infections. Women with this condition often experience bladder and vaginal infections.

If any of these symptoms manifest on a regular or unusual basis, it is time to see a doctor, who can perform routine diabetes tests. We'll cover more on this in a later section of this chapter.

TESTS & DIAGNOSIS

A routine diabetes screening can diagnose Type II diabetes. Once the diagnosis is determined, your doctor will instruct you about closely following his advice (medical, holistic, or laser) until your blood sugar level drops and stabilizes.

Tests used to diagnose Type II diabetes are:

- HbA1C test has become the standard test for diagnosing diabetes. HbA1C is a glycated hemoglobin (A1C) test, which indicates your average blood sugar level for the past two or three months. HbA1C is considered the most accurate test to positively diagnose diabetes. This is determined by measuring the percentage of blood sugar attached to hemoglobin, the oxygen-carrying protein in red blood cells. The higher your blood sugar levels, the more sugar-attached hemoglobin you will have. The American Diabetic Association recommends an HbA1C of 7 percent or less and the American Society of Clinical Endocrinologists recommends 6.5 percent or less.

- Random plasma glucose test (also known as the casual plasma glucose test), in which a blood sample is taken at a random time. Regardless of when the person ate last, a random blood sugar level of 200 milligrams per deciliter (mg/dL) or higher suggests diabetes, particularly if the person experiences increased urination, increased thirst, and unexplained weight loss, as well as fatigue, blurred vision, cuts, and abrasions that do not heal, and increased hunger.

- Fasting plasma glucose (FPG) test, during which a blood sample is taken after fasting (no food for at least eight hours). Doctors prefer this diagnostic test, because it is convenient and inexpensive for the patient. Results are most reliable if the FPG test is taken in the morning. A fasting blood sugar level of 70 to 100 mg/dL is normal, whereas a level between 100 and 125 mg/dL indicates an increased risk of developing Type II diabetes, while a level of 126 mg/dL or higher on two separate tests is sufficient for a diagnosis of diabetes.

- The oral glucose tolerance test (OGTT), taken after a person has fasted for eight hours or more and two hours after the person has drunk 75 grams of glucose dissolved in water. This test, which is less convenient for the patient than the FPG test, can be used to diagnose both pre-diabetes and Type II diabetes. If the OGTT test shows a blood glucose level of 140 to 199 mg/dL, the diagnosis is considered to be impaired glucose tolerance (IGT), which is a form of pre-diabetes or an increased risk of developing Type II diabetes. If the blood glucose level is 200 mg/dL or higher, after a repeat test on another day, the diagnosis is diabetes.

The American Diabetes Association recommends adults, beginning at the age of forty-five, undergo routine screening for Type II diabetes, particularly if they are overweight and inactive. If the results are normal, the test should be repeated every three years; if borderline, it should be repeated annually.

SHORT-TERM COMPLICATIONS

Immediate medical attention is required if short-term complications, such as high blood sugar, increased ketones in your urine (see Point 2 below) or low blood sugar, arise. The risk of serious conditions (seizures and coma) increases if these complications are not addressed promptly or are left untreated.

1. **High blood sugar** (hyperglycemia). This complication occurs when you have eaten too much, have been sick, or have not taken the prescribed amount of glucose-lowering medication. It is important to check your blood sugar level often and monitor symptoms characteristic of hyperglycemia (frequent urination, increased thirst, dry mouth, blurred vision, fatigue, and nausea). To treat this problem, alter your meal plan or medications or both. Seek emergency care if your blood sugar level persistently goes above 250 mg/dL.

2. **Increased ketones** in urine (diabetic ketoacidosis). Ketones or toxic acids are the products of fat metabolism when your cells need energy. Symptoms of this complication are loss of appetite, nausea, vomiting, fever, stomach pain, and a sweet, fruity smell on your breath. These symptoms are more likely to be present if your blood sugar level consistently tests at 250 me/dL or higher. Excess ketones in your urine means you should seek emergency care or consult your physician.

3. **Low blood sugar** (hypoglycemia). Your blood sugar level can drop for any number of reasons, including skipping meals or being less active than normal; the problem is most likely if you take glucose-lowering medications that promote the insulin secretion or if you are undergoing insulin therapy. Early symptoms of low blood sugar include sweating, shakiness, weakness, hunger, dizziness, and nausea. Untreated, other symptoms may arise, such as slurred speech, drowsiness, and confusion. You can offset these symptoms by eating hard candy, a sweet snack or glucose tablets, or drinking juice or

regular soda to quickly raise your blood sugar level. If you lose consciousness, you will probably need an emergency injection of glucagon to stimulate the release of sugar into your bloodstream.

Long-Term Complications

Long-term complications develop gradually, but the earlier you are diagnosed with Type II diabetes and the less your blood sugar is controlled, the greater your risk of getting diabetes and, over time, may become disabling or life-threatening. Some long-term complications are:

- **Kidney damage (nephropathy).** The millions of tiny blood vessel clusters that make up your kidneys filter out waste from your blood. Diabetes can damage this filtering system, and if the damage is severe, it can lead to kidney failure or irreversible end-stage kidney disease that requires dialysis or a kidney transplant. *Diabetes is the leading cause of kidney failure. An estimated 44 million people are on kidney dialysis.* Note the N of 1 study discussed in a later chapter. The kidneys had failed and this man was on dialysis for five hours twice a week. He reversed the kidney damage and avoided a kidney transplant with QLaser therapy.

- **Alzheimer's disease.** The risk of this complication grows in relation to your blood sugar control. It is theorized that the cardiovascular problems caused by diabetes may contribute to dementia by blocking blood flow to the brain or causing strokes. Tight "dental muscles" also reduce blood glucose to the brain and are frequently overlooked in Alzheimer's. It is also possible that too much insulin in the blood leads to brain-damaging inflammation; conversely, lack of insulin in the brain can deprive its cells of glucose.

- **Eye damage.** Type II diabetes can damage the blood vessels of the retina (diabetic retinopathy) and eventually lead to blindness. It also increases the risk of developing cataracts and glaucoma. *Diabetes is the leading cause of new cases of blindness among adults aged twenty to seventy-four years.*

- **Foot problems.** Poor blood circulation or nerve damage in the feet increases the risk of a number of complications. Serious infections can result from untreated cuts and blisters, and in severe cases, such damage may necessitate amputation of a toe, foot, or even part of a leg. (Note the N of 1 study in a later chapter, where amputation of the toe was avoided with just three laser applications). *More than 60 percent of non-traumatic amputation of feet and legs occurs in people with diabetes. In 2004, that represents 71,000 amputations.*

- **Heart and blood vessel disease.** There is a dramatic increase in the risk of developing this long-term complication if you have Type II diabetes. Problems in this category include coronary artery disease with chest pain (angina), heart attack, stroke, narrowing of the arteries (atherosclerosis), and high blood pressure. According to a study in 2007, the risk of stroke more than doubles within the first five years of being treated for Type II diabetes, and about 75 percent of people who have diabetes die of a heart or blood vessel disease. To make matters worse, many of the drugs that are prescribed for Diabetes Mellitus end up causing heart problems.

- **Nerve damage (neuropathy).** An excessive amount of sugar in the blood can damage the walls of tiny blood vessels (capillaries) that feed your nerves, particularly in the legs; the result can be tingling, numbness, burning, or pain. Usually the sensations begin in the toes or fingers and spread upward over a period of time; untreated, you could lose all sensation in the affected limbs. When there is damage to nerves that control digestion, you could experience nausea, vomiting, diarrhea, or constipation. Erectile dysfunction is an additional problem for men. *Between 60 and 70 percent of diabetics have mild to severe forms of nervous system damage, resulting in impaired sensation or pain in feet or hands, slowed digestion in the stomach, carpel tunnel syndrome, and other problems?*

- **Osteoporosis.** The presence of diabetes may lead to lower bone density, which increases the risk of your developing osteoporosis.

- **Skin and mouth conditions.** With diabetes, skin problems, such as bacterial or fungal infections and itching, as well as gum infections, particularly if you have a history of poor dental hygiene, may arise. *Periodontal or gum disease is more common in diabetics; almost a third of diabetics have severe gum disease.*

Type II diabetes is manageable—and even preventable—but you must be fully aware of the signs and symptoms and possible short-term and long-term complications in order to address them promptly and properly.

TYPE II DIABETES AND DEPRESSION

According to a five-center study released by Sherita Hill Golden, MD, of Johns Hopkins, and colleagues in the June 18, 2008 issue of the *Journal of the American Medical Association*, there is a correlation between patients with Type II diabetes and depression; they are more likely to develop depression. They found that "patients under treatment for Type II diabetes, but not those with untreated disease of comparable severity, were at a significantly increased risk for developing depressive symptoms over the next few years."

They suggested that the "worries and burdens of managing their diabetes may lead to depression" and that "the psychological stress associated with diabetes management may lead to elevated depressive symptoms."

Study investigators found an insignificant trend for depressed patients to develop Type II diabetes; the disease may have developed "primarily because of lifestyle changes engendered by depression." Dr. Golden and colleagues recommended that clinicians consider screening their Type II diabetes patients for depressive symptoms, because depressed patients are less likely to comply with dietary and weight loss recommendations and are more likely to be physically inactive.

ACCELERATING COSTS

The direct and indirect costs of treating diabetes and its attendant healthcare problems in the United States are staggering. In 2007, the total annual economic cost of diabetes, according to the American Diabetes Association (ADA), was approximately $174 billion. This figure was first reported in a study done with the ADA and Novo Nordisk, the world's top producer of insulin and diabetes pills (NovoNorm and Prandin).

Direct medical expenditures were $116 billion, and the breakdown was as follows:

- $27 billion for diabetes care

- $58 billion for chronic diabetes-related complications

- $31 billion for excess general medical costs.

Indirect costs resulting from increased absenteeism, reduced productivity, disease-related unemployment disability, and loss of productive capacity due to early mortality carried a hefty price tag, as well: $58 billion, an increase of $42 billion since 2002. Translated, this 32 percent increase means the dollar amount has increased each year by $8 billion.

A new study, conducted by the Lewin Group and released in 2008, revealed a total of $218 billion for 2007 in direct medical care costs from insulin and drugs to amputations and hospitalization, plus indirect costs, such as lost productivity, disability, and early retirement. This study adds estimates for people not yet been diagnosed ($18 billion), women who develop gestational diabetes ($636 million), and those with the likelihood of developing diabetes (pre-diabetics) at $25 billion.

"This study gives a very persuasive argument to employers to invest in a culture of health in their workforce," said Andrew Webber, president and chief executive of the National Business Coalition on Health. He called the worsening diabetes epidemic "the tsunami that is coming."

It may seem strange to you that I wait until the end to tell you how easy it is to treat diabetes with the QLaser System and how much money it will save, but first I will discuss the conventional treatments and horrendous costs of treating diabetes. While it should be obvious that one should try to prevent the onset of diabetes, prevention will be discussed in Chapter 3, along with alternative treatments of Type II diabetes. Beyond that, we will discuss the low level laser and the benefits it delivers in diabetes and in the healthcare arena.

DID YOU KNOW?

- Type II diabetes is the most frequent condition in people with kidney failure in Western countries.

- Diabetes is the largest cause of kidney failure in developed countries, resulting in spiraling dialysis costs.

- The risk for death among people with diabetes is about twice that of people without diabetes of similar age.

- Diabetes was the seventh leading cause of death listed on U.S. death certificates in 2006.

- Diabetes is underreported as cause of death; only 35 to 40 percent list it on the death certificate and far less listed it as underlying cause of death.

- Ten percent to 20 percent of diabetics die of renal failure.

- Every ten seconds, a person dies from diabetes-related causes.

- One out of every five healthcare dollars is spent caring for someone with diagnosed diabetes.

Chapter 2

Conventional Treatments

Half the modern drugs
could well be thrown out
the window, except that
the birds might eat them.

Martin H. Fischer

The failure of the U.S. medical system in providing decent medical care for Americans remains stunning, if not alarming. The fact that the medical system itself has played a large role in undermining the health of Americans is shameful, indeed.

In an article published in the *Journal of the American Medical Association (JAMA)*, several research studies in the previous decade revealed that 225,000 Americans died as a result of medical treatments—or should we say mistreatments—as follows:

- 12,000 deaths per year due to unnecessary surgery

- 7,000 deaths per year due to medication errors in hospitals

- 20,000 deaths per year due to other hospital errors

- 80,000 deaths per year due to infections in hospitals

- 106,000 deaths per year due to negative effects of drugs.

America's healthcare-system-induced deaths are the third leading cause of death in the U.S., after heart disease and cancer. In reality, many deaths are attributed to heart attack, but the drugs are what triggered the heart attack.

"The traditional medical paradigm that emphasized the use of prescription medicine and medical treatment has not only failed to improve the health of Americans, but it has also led to the decline in the overall well-being of Americans," said Barbara Starfield, MD, author of the article.

According to an article published in *Litigation/Medical Malpractice*, August 9, 2004, deaths from medical errors in U.S. hospitals were running at approximately 195,000 per year. HealthGrades, the healthcare quality company, released a study with some alarming findings:

- About 1.4 million patient-safety incidents occurred among the 37 million hospitalizations in the Medicare population over the years 2000 to 2002.

- Of the total 323,993 deaths among Medicare patients in those years that developed one or more patient-safety incidents, 263,864, or 81 percent, of these deaths were attributable to the incident(s).

- One in every four Medicare patients who were hospitalized from 2000 to 2002 experienced a patient-safety incident died.

- Patient-safety incidents with the highest rates per 1,000 hospitalizations were (1) failure to rescue patients from complications that can be fatal (also known as errors of omission); (2) decubitus ulcer, also known as bed sores, that is caused by poor blood circulation, resulting from excessive period of time that the hospital patient is not turned (cured with low level laser); (3) sepsis, a very serious, sometimes life-threatening infection following surgery that requires urgent health care intervention; these accounted for almost 60 percent of all patient-safety incidents.

- Overall, the best performing hospital (those with the lowest overall patient-safety incident rates, defined as the top 7.5 percent of all hospitals studied) had five fewer deaths per 1,000 hospitalizations compared to the bottom tenth percentile.

- Fewer patient-safety incidents in the best performing hospitals resulted in a lower cost of $740,337 per 1,000 hospitalizations, compared to the bottom tenth percentile of hospitals.

"If the Center for Disease Control's annual list of leading causes of death included medical errors, it would show up as Number 6, ahead of diabetes, pneumonia, Alzheimer's disease, and renal failure," noted Dr. Collier of HealthGrades. "Hospitals need to act on this, and consumers need to arm themselves with enough information to make quality-oriented health care choices when selecting a hospital."

Patients in the highest-rated, five-star hospitals in the United States are at a 65 percent lower chance of dying than patients in the lowest-rated, one-star hospitals, according to the 8th Annual HealthGrades Hospital Quality Study in America, released in October 2005 by HealthGrades, a healthcare ratings company.

If all hospitals included in the study performed at the five-star level, more than 273,000 Medicare patients would have been saved in just 2002 to 2004, based on 37 million Medicare hospital records. Fifty percent of those potentially preventable deaths were associated with four diagnoses: heart failure, community-acquired pneumonia, sepsis, and respiratory failure.

The study found a growing "quality chasm." While overall death rates at hospitals improved 12 percent, the best-performing hospitals lowered their death rates 45 percent faster than the lowest-ranking hospitals. Reasons given include high hospital volumes and more physicians who specialize in the critically ill.

With these stunning facts, anyone seeking medical care takes a risk; with Type II diabetes patients, the risk is compounded when their doctors prescribe pharmaceutical drugs that carry dangerous, even lethal, side effects. Many of the studies quoted here are eight to ten years old, and statistics are worse today—not better. We will discuss side effects of drugs later.

TREATMENTS

Conventional treating Type II diabetes requires a serious commitment to monitoring blood sugar, following a healthy diet, exercising regularly, and, if strictly following conventional treatment, taking diabetes medications or undergoing insulin therapy. The overall goal is to maintain your blood sugar level as normal as possible to offset complications, such as heart disease, strokes, and blindness. With proper, strict control of your blood sugar levels, you can reduce the risk of these complications by more than 50 percent. Treating with low level laser will be discussed later.

Like most stressful problems we face in life, it is best to deal with them a day at a time. Millions of people are in the same boat, and since Type II diabetes is a familiar health problem, there are ample healthcare professionals, educators, and diet specialists that can provide proper treatment guidelines to help you reach your goal.

First and foremost is monitoring your blood sugar level as often as daily or at least several times a week. Your physician will set a target range; careful monitoring will help you keep your blood sugar within that range. The biggest problem is that the amount of sugar in your blood can change erratically, even if you are watching your diet carefully. Your physician and other healthcare professionals will teach you how blood sugar levels vary with the following:

- **Food.** Your food choices affect your blood sugar level, which is usually highest an hour or two after eating a meal. *Intolerant or allergic foods are as bad as or worse than high sugar foods.*

- **Exercise**. The more active you are, the more sugar you move from your blood into your cells

- **Medication**. Your medications are designed to help you control your blood sugar levels, but sometimes they need to be changed or eliminated or your overall treatment plan may need to be altered. The side effects of medication should be of major concern. Medications differ for different people.

- **Illness**. Hormones produced by your body to fight a cold or other illness raise your blood sugar level

- **Alcohol.** Depending on when you drink or if you drink and eat at the same time, alcohol can cause either high blood sugar or low blood sugar

- **Stress**. In response to stress, your body produces hormones, which prevent insulin from working properly. Hidden stress or Dental Distress Syndrome is present in nearly every diabetic and is a major contributor to an imbalance in the autonomic nervous system (ANS).

- **Hormone level fluctuation** (in women). During menstrual cycles, your blood sugar level may fluctuate, and later in life, menopause can do the same.

In the beginning, daily blood sugar monitoring is important to help you understand how any of the above can affect your levels, but your doctor may also want you to undergo regular PbA1C testing to determine your average blood sugar levels for the past two or three months. This is a better indicator than daily testing about how well your treatment plan is working. A spike in your PbA1C level may require a change in your treatment plan, either in medication or diet. As you will learn later, low level laser therapy lowers HBA1C.

Eating Healthy

The same healthy diet you follow to *prevent* diabetes is very similar to the one you would follow to *treat* the condition. Eating plenty of fruits (with some restrictions, such as melons, due to their high sugar content), vegetables (again with similar restrictions for high-sugar vegetables like corn and peas), whole grains (no white flour products, such as bread and pasta), and limiting animal products will give you a wide variety, so you won't get bored.

Some diabetes specialists adhere to stricter dietary guidelines than others, but the American Diabetes Association recommends a food exchange program that allows diabetics to enjoy a sweet treat now and then, as long as they include it in their regular meal plan. The main concerns are to carefully watch their carbohydrates, proteins, fat, and calories; be consistent in planning meals; and eat several small meals a day in order to maintain a balanced blood sugar level.

There is increasing interest in food intolerances and food allergies and the effect they have on diabetes. Intolerant or allergic reactions spike blood sugar rapidly. There are many ways of testing for these conditions which are commonly missed, but a favorite is the Elisa/Act blood test.

EXERCISING REGULARLY

Just as daily exercise is a good preventive routine, it is very important if you have been diagnosed with diabetes, if your doctor approves. You might have to start slowly if you led a sedentary life for awhile, but you can go for a walk or ride your bike or swim a few laps every day, until you build up your ability to exercise for thirty minutes or more several days a week. Exercise, in combination with a sound diet, lowers blood sugar. It is important to have a snack and check your blood sugar before you exercise, so your sugar level doesn't drop too much during exercise.

TAKING MEDICATIONS OR FOLLOWING INSULIN THERAPY

It is possible for diabetics to use diet and exercise to manage their blood sugar, but some on conventional therapy will need medications or insulin therapy to accomplish the same goal. This book offers low level laser therapy as an alternate to those sometimes dangerous and expensive drugs. Type II diabetics, through their physician, have a choice of different medications—some oral and some by injection. The choice depends on the need to stimulate the pancreas to produce and release more insulin; to stem the production and release of glucose from the liver; or to block stomach enzymes from breaking down carbohydrates or making the body's tissues more sensitive to insulin. Some physicians also prescribe low-dose aspirin therapy to prevent heart and blood vessel disease.

Insulin therapy (injections) might be necessary for some Type II diabetics, because their stomach enzymes interfere with insulin taken orally. There are several types of insulin, some that act quickly, while others are made to last over a longer period of time. After careful instructions and practice, most diabetics have no problem administering their own injections of insulin, using a fine needle and syringe or similar device.

Your blood sugar level and other health problems will help your doctor determine which medications and/or which type of insulin to use, and together you will monitor your sugar to see if alternations in your overall treatment plan are warranted.

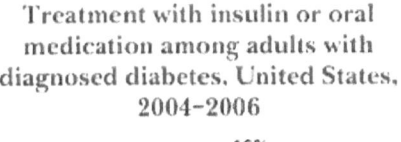

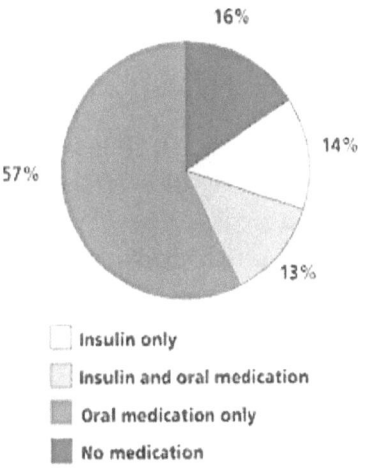

Source: 2004-2006 National Health Interview Survey

U.S. HEALTHCARE SYSTEM FAILURES

One doesn't have to look far to find yet another misstep in the American medical and pharmaceutical industries. Malpractice and class action lawsuits abound, and the cost of supporting the system continues to wreak havoc on our economy. Headlines call attention to negligence by healthcare practitioners, dangerous side effects of drugs, and even deaths caused by both.

For many years now, the life expectancy ranking for the United States has slipped behind that of forty-one other countries that have decreased the emphasis on diagnosis, improved healthcare delivery, and succeeded in encouraging their citizens to adopt healthier diets and lifestyles. Bureaucratic red tape hinders access to valuable therapies in the United States, forcing Americans to seek medical care overseas, in Canada, or in Mexico.

The American pharmaceutical industry, together with the Food &

Drug Administration, has a history of releasing medications that, after a period of time in use by consumers, must be withdrawn due to extreme complications, even death. Drugs, once approved by the FDA, are routinely recalled in the face of these complications, causing approvals of new drugs to dip significantly. Drugs designed to cure one problem often open up a Pandora's Box of side effects worse than the condition the drugs aim to correct in the first place. Avandia a common drug prescribes for Diabetes Mellitus is and example. Avandia has been under fire since 2007 over concerns that it raises the risk of heart attack, stroke, and death.

According to a report released July 20, 2006 by the Institute of Medicine of the National Academies, medication errors harm at least 1.5 million people every year. The extra medical costs of treating drug-related injuries occurring in hospitals amounts to $3.5 billion, conservatively speaking, not counting lost wages and productivity or additional health costs.

Four hundred thousand preventable drug-related injuries occur each year in hospitals, another 800,000 occur in long-term care facilities, and approximately 530,000 occur just among Medicare recipients in outpatient settings. The average resident of a nursing care facility takes nine drugs per day—many that cause side reactions that complicate and exacerbate reactions of other drugs.

Confusion caused by drugs with similar names accounts for 25 percent or so of all errors. Labeling and packaging cause 33 percent of errors, including 30 percent of all related fatalities.

THE DRAWBACKS OF ANTI-DIABETES DRUGS

Really there are no sage drugs. On the other hand, low level laser therapy is completely safe and has no interaction with other drugs or medications.

According to *Consumer Reports*, there are six types (eleven individual drugs) or oral medicines on the market to help millions of Type II diabetics control their blood sugar when diet and lifestyle changes cannot sufficiently do so. According to the publication's report, updated in February 2009, some interesting facts emerged:

- Newer drugs are no better than those that had been on the market for years, even decades. (Two drugs classified as sulfonylureas and Metformin have been available for more than a decade and work as well as newer drugs. And, as you will read in this chapter, some of the newer drugs have proven to be less effective and less safe than the older ones.)

- Newer drugs offer no greater safety than older ones; in fact, all anti-diabetes medications carry the potential to trigger side effects, some serious. It is therefore vital to check the safety profile of any drug in this category before taking it.

- Newer drugs are more expensive, often many times more so than the older ones.

- While it is sometimes necessary to take more than one diabetes drug, taking more than one raises the risk of adverse side effects, drug interactions, and increases costs.

Therefore, considering effectiveness, safety, side effects, dosing, and costs— and considering that the recommended drugs are available in low-cost generic form, *Consumer Reports* makes the following recommendations:

- Metformin, alone or with glipizide or glimepiride

- Glipizide & Glipizide Sustained Release—alone or with Metformin

- Glimepiride—alone or with Metformin

METFORMIN

First marketed in the U.S. by Bristol-Myers Squibb in March 3, 1995, Metformin is the diabetes medication with the longest history in the U.S. and is the preferred oral drug for treatment of Type II diabetes, especially for those who are overweight or obese and those with normal kidney function.

In 2006, more than 35 million prescriptions for Metformin were written, and those were just for generic Metformin. Let's do the math, and this math could be done for each diabetic drug and insulin. A one-month prescription for Metformin costs around $20—that's $140 a year or 420 million a year spent by just three million of the US's approximately twenty million acute diabetics. And that doesn't include the cost of other medical conditions caused by the diabetes plus the risk of the drug side effects. I ask you the question: doesn't a non-prescription, low level laser make more economic sense?

According to numerous studies of Metformin, the most common side effects are: diarrhea (53.2 percent of people), nausea or vomiting (25.5 percent), flatulence (gas) (12.1 percent), weakness (9.2 percent), indigestion (7.1 percent), abdominal discomfort (6.4 percent), and headache (5.7 percent).

BYETTA

Byetta, a unique FDA-approved medicine, helps treat people with Type II diabetes in a different way than other drugs or insulin. Byetta helps the body produce the right amount of insulin at the right time. In doing so, the person feels less hungry and eats less, enjoying a positive side effect: weight loss. Byetta is not a weight-loss drug, but one study of Byetta in patients showed that, on average, they lost five pounds over a thirty-week period.

The drug comes in pre-measured, easy-to-use dosage pens, which makes it convenient to use anywhere without having to measure. Patients see improved blood glucose levels as early as Day One.

Not all anti-diabetes drugs can paint as rosy a picture as Metformin and Byetta. Some drugs, in fact, have been recalled due to serious adverse effects, even death. Let's look at three of those drugs: Avandia, Rezulin, and Tequin.

AVANDIA

A year later, in October 2008, Public Citizen, a consumer group, petitioned the Food & Drug Administration to withdraw Avandia and ban its use, due to life-threatening risks, including heart and liver damage. The manufacturer, GlaxoSmithKline, had already suffered a setback when the American Diabetes Association and its European counterpart called for a similar ban on the drug.

"The FDA is in possession of clear, unequivocal evidence that [Avandia] causes a wide variety of toxicities," Public Citizen said in its petition. "Many of these are life-threatening, such as heart attacks, heart failure and liver failure."

Two years earlier, an article in a medical journal cited a 43 percent greater risk of heart attacks among patients using Avandia, compared to patients taking other diabetes medications. The scientific debate continues, and the FDA continues to monitor Avandia's safety record, but the concerns about the medical evidence have led to stronger warnings, resulting in a sharp drop in the use of Avandia; however, even after all of these warnings, approximately one million patients continue to take the drug.

Research by Public Citizen discovered fourteen cases of liver failure associated with Avandia, and twelve of them led to death. The petition also cited predisposition to eye problems, anemia, and bone fractures in patients using Avandia.

In addition to liver failure, the following safety concerns were cited:

- **Myocardial ischemia**, also known as angina, a painful heart condition due to a temporary lack of oxygen to the heart—a 40 percent increase in the risk of heart attacks

- **Congestive heart failure**, which results when the heart can no longer pump enough blood to other organs—the risk of this complication is doubled

- **Macular edema**, a swelling or thickening of the macula, the small area in the center of the retina that allows one to see fine articles clearly; caused by leaking from retinal blood vessels— the rate was thirty times higher than with other drugs

- **Anemia**, the most common blood disorder which is a decrease in the normal number of red blood cells—consistently associated with usage of Avandia.

- **Fractures** – Avandia negatively affects bone density.

A British study released in December of 2008 and published in the Canadian Medical Association Journal online revealed that two anti-diabetic drugs, Avandia and Actos, double the risk of fractures in women. Studies showed that these drugs reduced bone density in the spine and hips, doubling the risk of women to experience bone density loss or osteoporosis if a woman is already at risk for fractures, the study estimated the occurrence of one fracture for every twenty-one women.

While it is interesting to note that the same problem does not occur in men, the study group speculated that the problem in women is related to an interaction between the drugs and estrogen, which also weaken bones in women. It doesn't take much loss of bone mass to increase the risks of fractures, especially in women who have smaller, thinner bones.

Although approximately four million Americans take these drugs, women were cautioned to consider other drugs, due to heightened risks for heart failure, death, and heart attacks with Avandia. "The U.S. Food & Drug Administration needs to give a much stronger warning to women," said Dr. Yoon Loke, lead researcher of the Canadian study. "And the warning should be that really these drugs should be avoided, if at all possible."

In November 2008, the FDA *ordered a black box put on Avandia,* warning that the drug may cause myocardial infarction; it also called for extensive long-term trials to determine the drugs safety with relation to cardiovascular disease. The FDA also requested that GlaxoSmithKline compare Avandia to other approved oral diabetes drugs in large, lengthy cardiovascular outcomes studies, with periodic assessments.

BLACK BOX WARNING—AVANDIA

This black box warning is in addition to one that already addresses heart failure. The FDA also asked manufacturers of all oral diabetes medications to add the following language to their drug labels:

> *A meta-analysis of 42 clinical studies (mean duration six months; 14,237 total patients), most of which compared Avandia to placebo, showed Avandia to be associated with an increased risk of myocardial ischemic events such as angina or myocardial infarction. Three other studies (mean duration 41 months; 14,067 patients), comparing Avandia to some other approved oral anti-diabetic agents or placebo, have not confirmed or excluded this risk. In their entirety, the available data on the risk of myocardial ischemia are inconclusive. To date, no oral anti-diabetes drug has been conclusively shown to reduce cardiovascular risk.*

Due to health and safety concerns over the use of Avandia, in just a two-year period, U.S. prescriptions plummeted from a high of 3.5 million per quarter to 0.9 million per quarter in October 2008. This is just the latest in a series of missteps with anti-diabetes drugs.

REZULIN

The British recalled the diabetes drug, Rezulin, late in 1997, but the FDA in the United States waited for three years for safety checks on newer diabetes drugs. That's interesting, when you consider that Dr. Sidney Wolfe, long-time consumer advocate with Public Citizen, once described Rezulin as "one of the most dangerous drugs on the market." The FDA's delay in recalling the drug was, according to Wolfe, "another example of how low the standards have gotten at FDA."

As it was, Rezulin was railroaded through the FDA (or to put it more politely, its approval came on a fast-track period of just six months). At the time, it was the only drug that restored the body's sensitivity to insulin, which is at the heart of diabetes. Considered a "miracle drug" at the beginning, some diabetics were able to stop their insulin injections.

However, from the onset of consumer usage, reports of liver failure arose, and instead of immediately recalling the drug, the FDA ordered the manufacturer, Warner-Lambert, to issue stronger liver toxicity warnings on the drug label. Approximately two million people used Rezulin, despite those warnings, but when sixty-three people died of liver failure, the FDA finally agreed that Rezulin posed an "unacceptable risk to patients." There were twenty deaths in the first six weeks' of usage. Overall, 391 deaths were possibly linked to Rezulin. Some of the deaths were due to heart failure, another serious risk covered up by the pharmaceutical company.

The FDA itself eventually concluded that Rezulin patients were 1,200 times more likely to suffer liver failure, which, as the disease progresses, presents such possible side effects as:

- Coughing up or vomiting large amounts of blood

- Muscle wasting

- Jaundice

- Salivary gland enlargement

- Weakness

- Fatigue

- Weight loss

- Poor appetite

- Abdominal pain

- Nausea

- Fever

- Dark urine

- Shrinking testicles or enlarged male breasts

- Spider veins

- Hair loss

- Curling up of the fingers

- Redness of the palms

In more than three years that Rezulin was on the market, Warner-Lambert raked in $2.1 billion in sales. Countless lawsuits put a dent in their profits. As it turns out, Warner-Lambert knew about at least twelve people who suffered liver damage as early as 1993 during preliminary trials, but the manufacturer ignored this potential danger. "…approving drugs too readily and waiting too long to remove them…makes some people lose faith in the FDA," said Wolfe. "It also winds up killing a lot of people that wouldn't have been killed, had the drugs not been put on the market in the first place."

TEQUIN

Sometimes a drug is recalled, or the manufacturer stops making the drug, because one of the side effects is that it spikes the incidence of developing diabetes. Bristol-Meyers Squibb received a license to manufacture Tequin from a Japanese pharmaceutical company, and the FDA approved the antibiotic in 1999. The drug was primarily used to treat upper respiratory infections.

Early in 2006, rumors circulated that a Canadian study would be released that documented a high incidence of diabetes in patients taking Tequin. Prior to that study appearing in *The New England Journal of Medicine*, Bristol-Meyers Squibb decided to reveal some of the findings to doctors prescribing the drug. The FDA also added a black box warning.

It was too little, too late. Consumer outcry and publication of the Canadian study and others forced the company to stop manufacturing Tequin.

AGGRESSIVE GLUCOSE-LOWERING TREATMENT

In February 2008, the U. S. government and its National Heart, Lung & Blood Institute decided to drop their aggressive glucose-lowering strategy in Type II diabetics eighteen months early, due to its association with excess mortality. The study of 10,000 patients was ended, following 257 deaths that occurred in the group receiving intensive treatment, as opposed to 203 deaths in the standard-treatment group. All of the excess deaths were cardiovascular.

The aggressive approach used a mixture of drugs, including insulin and Avandia, as well as behavior modification, to treat patients. The conclusion reached was that high-risk diabetics—particularly older ones who have had diabetes for a longer period of time but who have poor glucose control and multiple risk factors—should be treated more conservatively.

The bigger problem is that, like typical conventional treatments, the focus is on fixing the symptom and not the underlying disease. For diabetics, treatments that concentrate just on lowering blood sugar, while raising insulin levels, can have disastrous results by worsening the problem of metabolic miscommunication.

THE HAZARDS OF DIABETES DRUGS

Most drugs used for treating Type II diabetics do one of two things: (1) raise insulin or (2) lower blood sugar. All this contributes to advancing side effects and shortening the diabetic's lifespan.

Diabetic drugs *don't work*, because they lower blood sugar by *increasing* fat cells at a faster pace; if sugar levels are lowered without converting them to energy, they convert to fat and cholesterol, causing the patient to gain weight. You see, these drugs are designed to multiply fat cells. There is no drug that works at the cell membrane level to allow insulin to enter the cell so that the cell can make ATP.

Low level laser therapy works by increasing nitric oxide levels, which carry insulin into the cells, and there are no side effects.

When a diabetic patient takes these drugs, instead of *reducing* their consumption of sugar, they are consuming too much, which turns to fat. All fat needs to be stored somewhere, and in this case, the patient ends up adding excess storage space, further complicating the problem. Eventually those fat cells become resistant to insulin, and the diabetic is back at the beginning of his or her problem. Conventional medicine then instructs the patient to simply increase the dosage! It's a never-ending cycle of health problems!

Is it any wonder why conventional medicine is going the way of covered wagons? In the next chapter, we share some encouraging and interesting alternative approaches to treating diabetes.

DID YOU KNOW?

- Every year 3.8 million deaths are attributable to diabetes worldwide, similar to the number of deaths due to HIV/AIDS. Even more die from cardiovascular disease, complicated by diabetes.

- Diabetes is the fourth leading cause of global death by disease.

- On average, people with Type II diabetes will die five to ten years before people without diabetes, mostly due to cardiovascular disease.

- People with Type II diabetes are as likely to suffer a heart attack as are people without diabetes who have already had a heart attack.

CHAPTER 3

HOLISTIC TREATMENTS

He's the best physician who knows
the worthlessness of most medicines.

Benjamin Franklin

Modern medicine, with the hundreds of billions of dollars spent on research, still has not made much headway in finding the cause of or treatment for the top diseases facing Americans today. How can this be? In a country that spends more money per capita, has more doctors, nurses, and lab technicians per capita, runs more laboratory tests, does more physical therapy, prescribes more drugs, and has more hospitals and nursing homes per capita than any other country in the world, why are we not at the top in health and happiness?

How can the United States produce such dismal statistics as these, the ten leading causes of death (as of 2006), based on the 2.4 million deaths, as reported by the Centers for Disease Control and Prevention?

1. Diseases of the heart – 631,250 or 26.3 percent of all deaths

2. Malignant neoplasm (cancer) – 559,804 or 23.3 percent

3. Cerebrovascular diseases (including the common stroke) – 136,976 or 5.7 percent

4. Chronic lower respiratory diseases (including emphysema and chronic bronchitis) – 124,549 or 5.2 percent

5. Unintentional injuries (accidents) – 120,395 or 5.0 percent

6. Diabetes Mellitus – 72,442 or 3.0 percent

7. Alzheimer's disease – 72,432 or 3.0 percent

8. Influenza and pneumonia – 56,060 or 2.3 percent

9. Nephritis (diseases affecting the kidneys) – 45,182 or 1.9 percent

10. Septicemia (resulting from infections in blood – virus, bacteria or fungus – occurring when a skin wound is not treated) – 33,965 or 1.4 percent

This list has not changed much in the past several decades, except for an increase in deaths from hospital and doctor-related causes and from Alzheimer's; both of these categories have increased dramatically.

The numbers are a bit misleading for deaths due at least in part to diabetes. According to death certificate reports, there were 233,619 deaths in 2005, for which the *contributing cause* of death was diabetes. Diabetes is not likely to be reported as a *cause* of death; in fact, only 35 to 40 percent of the deaths involving diabetes had it listed on the death certificate, and only 10 to 15 percent listed it as the *underlying cause* of death.

HEALTH RANKING

Why, in a country where we seem to have the most of everything, our current economic hardships, are we so sick and unhappy? Of the most economically advanced free world countries, the United States ranks near the bottom in health and longevity.

WHO World Health Report
Ranking the World's Health Systems 2000

France	Switzerland
Italy	Belgium
San Marino	Colombia
Andorra	Sweden
Malta	Cyprus
Singapore	Germany
Spain	Saudi Arabia
Oman	United Arab Emirates
Austria	Israel
Japan	Morocco
Norway	Canada
Portugal	Finland
Monaco	Australia
Greece	Chile
Iceland	Denmark
Luxembourg	Dominica
Netherlands	Costa Rica
United Kingdom	**United States**
Ireland	

Note: Due to the complexities of data gathering, this study has not been updated.

Note: In 2000, France ranked #1 and Italy #2; the United States lagged far behind at #37. More recently, an editorial in the August 12, 2007 edition of *The New York Times* cited the "disturbing truth" that the United States "lags well behind other advanced nations in delivering timely and effective healthcare." The editorial referred to the WHO ranking (previous page) and cited the May 2007 ranking of the highly regarded Commonwealth Fund that put the United States last or next-to-last, compared to Australia, Canada, Germany, New Zealand, and the United Kingdom in both quality of care and access to it.

THE RISE OF NATURAL MEDICINE

It should be no surprise why millions of Americans have turned to holistic, natural medicine, to alternative ways of treating whatever ails them.

The skyrocketing healthcare costs, coupled with the lack of affordable health insurance and the high cost of prescription medicine, have driven Americans to look to nature and to other cultures and times for home remedies. Americans are getting smarter. Just because insurance pays for something, they are not agreeing to the surgery, treatment, or the drugs. They are asking about risks, side effects, and wasting their insurance dollar; and more and more are turning to natural or energy medicine.

For the past twenty-five years, complementary, alternative, preventive or integrative medical groups have entered the healthcare field with high hopes of making a difference—changing the failed orthodox, conventional, western medicine model for health care, and educating people to use other methods in place of, or together with, conventional medicine. That goal is gradually being reached.

As of 2004, nearly half of all Americans have used at least one kind of complementary alternative medicine (CAM) at one time or another and more than 80 million were expected to use CAM that year. In 2006, over 50 percent of the 300 million U.S. residents used some type of integrative, complementary or alternative medicine; yet, at the same time, Americans have become sicker, more obese, and have died at younger ages. Obviously, something is missing.

Our healthcare systems are failing and have failed for some time, even after the general acceptance of preventive, alternative medicine. No politician can fix the healthcare dilemma we face today, and, in fact, many of the proposed laws take the responsibility of wellness away from the individual and place it under bureaucrats. Individuals, I maintain, must take responsibility for their own health, and not depend on others. They must stop overusing the system. The healthiest people use the system the least.

None of the sixty-seven specialties and subspecialties in the healthcare business in the U.S. is looking after the total being, and how the mind, body, and spirit function in the total health process. I contend that the specialty groups have overlooked or misunderstood two major factors that play a big role in the dismal state of health care in America.

We need to look at energy medicine, ancient Chinese medicine, Indian medicine, Middle Eastern medicine, and Native American medicine.

PREVENTION

The fastest way to eliminate the need for treatment is to prevent Type II diabetes in the first place. It all boils down to the choices one makes for a healthy lifestyle. Diabetes can be prevented, even if it runs in your family, or if you have already been diagnosed with this condition, by following these steps to help you avert some of the more serious complications, as discussed in Chapter 1:

1. Maintaining a healthy diet, low in fat and calories, and generous in fruits, vegetables, and whole grains.

2. Increasing your physical activity, at least half an hour a day, walking briskly, riding your bike, swimming laps, even in smaller time-sets will help you stay fit.

3. Shedding extra pounds, even as few as ten pounds, can make a difference in reducing the risk of diabetes.

4. Applying low level laser therapy on a preventive basis.

These four steps, when approached as permanent lifestyle changes or behavior modification, will not only lower your risk of a host of health problems, including diabetes, but will also give you more energy and greater self-esteem.

COMPLEMENTARY & ALTERNATIVE MEDICAL THERAPIES

According to the National Center for Complementary and Alternative Medicine, part of the National Institutes of Health, complementary and alternative medicine is a "group of diverse medical and healthcare systems, practices, and products that are not presently considered to be part of conventional medicine." Complementary medicine is used in conjunction with conventional treatments; alternative medicine is considered replacement therapy.

Patients with diabetes can use either complementary or alternative therapies for treatment, but it is important to understand that while some can be effective, others can be not only ineffective, but also harmful. It is therefore vital for patients to keep their healthcare providers informed of other therapies they undertake.

ACUPUNCTURE

In this ancient procedure, an acupuncture practitioner inserts needles into designated points on the patient's skin. Acupuncture, which some believe triggers release of the body's natural painkillers, is sometimes used by people with painful nerve damage due to diabetes.

According to traditional Chinese medicine, stress, trauma or other causes of emotional imbalance can be the cause or symptom of a disorder, such as diabetes. Diabetics often have nerve pain or uncomfortable nerve sensations that acupuncture can alleviate. Acupuncture releases muscle tension, allowing an increased flow of blood, lymph, and nerve impulses to affected areas.

In Chapter 7, I describe how traditional acupuncture can now be replaced by a low level laser stimulating acupuncture points with light, instead of puncturing them with a needle. This is particularly appealing to patients who are afraid of needles!

BIOFEEDBACK

This technique helps the diabetic patient become more aware of and learn to deal with the body's response to pain; the emphasis here is on techniques to relax and reduce stress. One relaxation technique is *guided imagery*, in which the patient thinks of peaceful mental images. Those who have used this technique believe their condition can be eased with these positive chronic disease-controlling images.

CHROMIUM

For several years, studies have been conducted and the benefits debated of adding chromium to the diet of diabetics. Chromium, which is needed to make glucose tolerance factor, helps insulin improve its action. However, despite the years of study and debate, there still is insufficient information on the use of chromium to recommend it as a supplement for treating diabetes.

GINSENG

Most studies of ginseng and diabetes have used American ginseng, and they have shown some glucose-lowering effects in fasting and after-meal blood glucose levels, as well as in A1C levels. More long-term studies are needed, however, before a general recommendation for use of ginseng in treating diabetes can be made; also, the amount of glucose-lowering compound in ginseng plants varies widely.

MAGNESIUM

The relationship between magnesium and diabetes has been studied for many years, but it still is not clearly understood. Some studies have shown that a magnesium deficiency may worsen blood glucose control in Type II diabetes. Scientists believe that such a deficiency interrupts insulin secretion in the pancreas and increases insulin resistance in the body's tissues. It may also contribute to certain diabetes complications.

People with higher dietary intakes of magnesium (through consumption of whole grains, nuts, and green leafy vegetables) have experienced a decreased risk of Type II diabetes.

VANADIUM

This compound, found in tiny amounts in plants and animals, has been shown to normalize blood glucose levels in animals with Type I and Type II diabetes. A recent study found that when diabetics were given vanadium, they developed a modest increase in insulin sensitivity and could decrease their insulin requirements. Researchers now want to understand how vanadium works in the body, study potential side effects, and determine safe dosages.

CINNAMON

Some studies have shown that cinnamon improves blood glucose control in people with Type II diabetes. In one study, sixty people with Type II diabetes were divided into six groups. Three groups took one, three or six grams of cinnamon per day, and the remaining groups took similar doses but of placebo capsules. After forty days, the groups that took all three doses of cinnamon realized significantly reduced fasting blood glucose, triglycerides, LDL cholesterol, and total cholesterol.

ZINC

Zinc is important for the production and storage of insulin. Some research shows that people with Type II diabetes have "suboptimal zinc status" due to decreased absorption and increased excretion of zinc.

NATURAL DIETARY REMEDIES

White is the "out" food. All of the foods we considered comfort foods when we were growing up—white bread, white pasta, white potatoes, white-sugar snacks, white-flour pastries—are on the DO NOT EAT list for Type II diabetics, mainly because they contain little or no fiber. Sugar, which comes disguised in a wide variety of pseudonyms, such as high fructose corn syrup (Public Enemy #1), robs our bodies of essential nutrients, and for the diabetic patient, sugar in all its forms should be avoided like the plague or, in some circumstances, consumed in greatly reduced amounts.

Removing or reducing consumption of processed and refined foods, which can rob you of nutrients and vitamins that your body needs to fend off stress and promote good health, is highly recommended. Foods in this category include fried foods, white pasta, white rice, full-fat dairy products, white potatoes, and white breads.

Instead, eat whole and unprocessed foods and avoid instant-type foods, preservatives, artificial flavors, saturated fats, hydrogenated foods, MSG, alcohol, and caffeine.

Other natural remedies for diabetes suggest that you:

- Adopt a high-fiber, high-complex carbohydrate diet distributed as follows: 60 percent carbohydrates, 20 percent proteins, and 20 percent fats.

- To keep blood sugar stable, eat six small meals a day with a higher good quality protein breakfast.

- Enjoy a midmorning and afternoon snack of fruit (i.e., an apple) to keep blood sugar stable.

- Adopt a regular exercise program.

- Make a serious attempt at controlling stress.(Read: *Healing Light* and concentrate on the chapters on Dental Distress Syndrome)

- Avoid emotional upsets, fatigue, and the use of tobacco.

Use of Herbal Products for Diabetes

Certified diabetes educators at The Cleveland Clinic have made the following recommendations for diabetic patients who are considering using herbal products as part of their treatment therapy:

- Discuss any drugs, including herbal products, with your doctor before taking them.

- If, as a result of taking an herbal product, you experience side effects, such as nausea, vomiting, rapid heartbeat, anxiety, insomnia, diarrhea, or skin rashes, stop taking the product and notify your physician immediately.

- Avoid preparations made with more than one herb; by using a one-herb product, you will be able to quickly determine if that particular herb produces negative side effects.

- Beware of "cure-all" commercial claims of herbal products. Check for scientific-based sources of information about the products and consult your physician before using them.

- Carefully select herbal brands and purchase only those that list the herb's common and scientific names, the name and address of the manufacturer, a batch and lot number, expiration date, dosage guidelines, and potential side effects.

Exercise and Diabetes

We have already discussed the problems that stress can cause for the diabetic patient. Here is good news: Exercise is one of the best ways to control stress. It can also be effective in preventing diabetes in the first place and in controlling blood sugar levels.

A study reported in *The New England Journal of Medicine* found that of the men involved in the study, those at highest risk of developing diabetes benefited the most from physical activity. Men who were very active and who burned 3,500 calories a week cut their risk of diabetes by half. Other studies have found that the same holds true for women, as well.

British researchers found that just seven minutes of exercise weekly may prevent diabetes by controlling blood sugar. However, the exercise must be vigorous, such as experienced in an all-out sprint. And all seven minutes do not have to be done at one time to be effective. In the study, volunteers rode exercise bikes four times per day in thirty-second spurts twice a week. After just two weeks, they had a 23 percent improvement in blood sugar control.

DID YOU KNOW?

- At least 50 percent of all people with diabetes are unaware of their condition. In some countries, that figure is as high as 80 percent.

- Up to 80 percent of Type II diabetes is preventable by adopting a healthy diet and increasing physical activity.

CHAPTER 4

ENERGY & LIGHT

*…happiness is the energy which
is the basis of health.*

Henri-Frédéric Amiel

Energy is eternal and omnipresent. Think of all the different kinds of energy that keep us and our world alive and moving forward. The energy of the universe maintains this magnificent globe, from solar energy to the energy imparted by the moon and ocean tides to energy derived from the wind and from the earth's natural resources.

Scientific research conducted over the past 300 years has revealed the importance of energy. Not only does everything we do depend on energy, but also everything on Earth, including human beings, *is* energy. Do you think a chair, for instance, is solid? Guess again. It is actually a manifestation of energy; we just don't see it in terms of energy because of the minute size of photons and atoms.

Harnessing energy for human use is not new. Think of all of our forerunners centuries ago that used the energy of their intellect and creativity to mastermind ways of using electricity (Benjamin Franklin, Nikla Tesla and others).

Many forms of powerful energy impact our everyday lives. We experience energy directly through our five senses. Our skin feels heat radiating from a fire. We feel forward motion when gravity causes our bicycle to accelerate when going downhill. We feel the force of kinetic energy when hammering a nail into a thick board. We feel the force of gravity when jumping up and down on a trampoline. From the force of energy, we hear the sound waves of someone's voice calling us.

Consider how we react to various forms of energy. Our eyes squint from bright sunlight after watching a movie for two hours in a darkened theater. We feel the shock of a small electric spark, as we walk across a carpet and then touch an object, such as a doorknob, a pet, or another person.

Everything we use in our daily lives comes about by the intricate use of energy in one way or another; yet, we are often unmindful of its role in affording us the conveniences we so enjoy, or we take it for granted. From the food we eat to the telephones we use to the cars we drive and the homes we heat and cool, energy is paramount in importance.

ENERGY IN MEDICINE

The use of energy in medicine is no exception. For many years now, medical science has applied laser energy to the healing process. Laser procedures for the treatment of hemorrhoids and for the correction of vision are two of the most widely used; both have achieved tremendous success. Without the use of lasers in these procedures and others, the recovery and rehabilitation would have been long, arduous, and often painful. Laser surgery has been a tremendous breakthrough in medicine.

LIGHT ENERGY

Light energy is the basis for all existence on planet Earth. It is no accident that the opening paragraph of the Bible describes the formation of the universe as beginning with light:

> In the beginning, God created the heaven and the earth. Now the earth was unformed and void, and darkness was upon the face of the deep; and the spirit of God hovered over the face of the waters. And God said, "Let there be light." And there was light. And God saw the light, that it was good.

In fact, there are more than 200 references to the word "light" in the Bible; seventy-five of them are in the New Testament.

Although early mankind lacked an understanding of science as we know it today, they recognized the fundamental importance of light energy. Thousands of years ago, they correlated the light of the moon and sun with crop planting and harvesting, for instance. The ancient Inca culture depended on light and may have used lasers powered by the sun to cut their sixty-ton stone blocks. Early astronomers learned the value of the sun, moon, and stars.

Think of the sun as an atomic furnace that turns mass into energy. Every fifteen minutes, the sun radiates as much energy as mankind consumes in all forms in an entire year, and the sun is 93 million miles from Earth!

The earth is awash in sunlight, which heats the earth's surface and atmosphere. Without sunlight, the earth would be a frozen rock floating in the dark, lifeless vacuum of space. The light itself is a force that makes life on earth possible. As seen from outer space, the green and blue earth bursts with life.

There would be no plant life without light and its stimulation of biological activity. Green plants depend entirely on photosynthesis for their metabolic processes. Once the seeds sprout forth, the life force of plants must have the energy of sunlight to continue; more specifically, plants require particular wavelengths of light, either natural or artificial. With a sufficient amount and type of light, green plants thrive. Without it, they dry up and die.

As with plant life, human cells require light energy. Light is crucial in the production of Vitamin D, essential for the metabolism of calcium and phosphorus. Without Vitamin D, our bones and muscles would suffer a variety of ailments (cramps, rheumatism, rickets, and tooth decay). Fortunately, Vitamin D is produced by the skin when it is exposed to the ultraviolet wavelengths of light contained in direct sunlight and in a tanning salon.

Although Vitamin D is in the food we eat, we can offset any possible deficiency, as long as we are exposed to an adequate amount of life-sustaining light from the sun.

Normally, the body must supply its own energy for metabolic activity, but what happens when the body has problems functioning, perhaps due to a serious injury or the advancing of old age? More raw materials for these chemical reactions can be supplied, but nutrients alone might not be able to speed up our metabolism. How can we add the energy that our cells need for chemicals to react faster?

Energy, energy, energy – it seems everyone today talks about energy, but what is energy? It is everywhere. Trucks run on it; airplanes fly on it;some people have "high energy"; the symphony or the basketball team played with great energy; there was great energy in the room; and it goes on and on. Books have been written about energy. So, what is "energy"? In the beginning, God saw the light, and it was good – then everything must be made of light. The fifth-century Greek philosophers, Democritus and Leucippus, first theorized atoms and said that everything in the universe of mass was composed of atoms.

An atom is a positive charge called the proton held together by a neutral charge called the neutron and a negative charge – the electron orbiting in some manner around the proton. The proton is very stable unless there is an atomic bomb or a hydrogen collider, but the electron is very elusive. The greatest physicists of the world do not know why the electron leaves the orbit around the proton. (Just a thought: If the greatest physicists do not know why the electron leaves and all cells are composed of atoms, how can doctors be so sure of the diagnosis of a disease?)

After decades of research dedicated to answering this question, I have developed a method of adding electrons (energy) to the body, which stimulates cellular activity. I have discovered that combined low level laser wavelengths, positioned to form soliton waves, powered correctly, and at specific frequencies, put electrons back at the atomic level. Atoms that lose electrons become ions, and ions are acid-forming, plus ions accelerate the redox mechanism causing accelerated oxidation and early cell death. Putting electrons back changes ions back to atoms, and stimulates metabolic processes at the cellular level. Yes, light can stimulate healing!

Before we delve more deeply into the healing power of light, let's take a look at the miracle of light itself.

LIGHT

Everything is defined by light; no object can be recognized in total darkness. Without light, there would be no life, which is dependent on three things: 1) the basic molecule-building block, carbon, 2) water, and 3) light. Earth has all three.

Light, therefore, is fundamental to our lives. Most of our knowledge of the world is based on our sight. Simply through observation, early humans tracked the cycles of natural events.

Lightning that set a bush or tree ablaze might well have been mankind's first introduction to fire, and early man then used campfires to liberate them from the cold and darkness of night and protect them from predators.

Four hundred thousand years ago, the first portable lamps were simple bundles of sticks tied together, but they enabled man to pursue activities at night or in dark caves.

From there, it was progression of discoveries and refinements to modern-day electric light. Archaeologists in France have discovered caves dating back 15,000 years, in which primitive lamps fashioned of shells, horns, rocks, and stones and filled with grease and using a fiber wick were found.

In ancient Egypt, light was a luxury. The pharaohs' palaces were illuminated only by the flickering flames of open bowls of animal fat, fish oil, or vegetable oil (palm and olive) with spouts to hold the wicks. In Ephesus, where Peter preached Christianity, the streets were lined with street lights of burning oil.

As man grew in knowledge of light and the energy it imparts, he used it in countless ways, from measuring time (early sundial) to entertaining (imagine watching one of Shakespeare's plays by candlelight).

Euclid, a Greek mathematician, concluded that the speed of light must be very high, because you can close your eyes (thus making the things you were looking at disappear), and when you open them again, even the distant stars appear instantly.

Pharaohs used fire at the top of the lighthouse that stood in the harbor of Alexandria, Egypt to signal ships on the Mediterranean; it was the archetype of every modern lighthouse.

Stonehenge, the monument of massive boulders erected in a circle by stone-age tribes in Great Britain, is aligned with planetary cycles and other astronomical events that those early people observed in the sky. Our ancestors were so intrigued with the sun, moon, and all the small lights they saw in the sky that they devoted their civilization to these natural spectacles. Without fully understanding what they were seeing, their confidence in what they observed inspired them to record their knowledge in stone for all time.

Light always comes from some particular source and direction. Throughout time, man has tried to understand the sun, moon, stars, and lightning. Benjamin Franklin supported the hypothesis that lightning was an electrical phenomenon. He not only explained positive and negative electricity; his work led to the development of the lightning rod. Today we all use Franklin's "electron – icity".

Nikla Tesla, an unsung hero in the field of energy, invented the generator for A/C (alternate current), which was at the center of the most basic decision about how to electrify America. While Edison, a genius in his own right, proposed to wire the country for D/C (direct current), he could not figure out a way to send high power across the distances that A/C could. Tesla, who started with Edison but turned aside monetary gain that would have come with work for corporations (he died broke in 1943), went on to invent the wireless radio and television, and a way to beam power (electrons) directly across the atmosphere.

Fascinated with lightning and electricity, Tesla held that Earth, rotating within the center of a magnetic field, was essentially a huge electrical generator. It is said that if Tesla were to come back from the dead, he would observe our current use of electricity and say, "You mean they make you pay for this?!"

Light stimulates the imagination and curiosity of not only scientists, but also artists and musicians. The French painter, Georges De La Tour, created works that always had pensive figures illuminated by a single candle, creating atmospheric extremes of light and darkness. The Dutch artist, Rembrandt, as a child, worked in a tall, dark windmill. Day after day, he sat and watched the rhythmic light, as the rotating arms of the windmill continuously flickered past one small window. Perhaps this early experience influenced the artist to create masterpieces that vibrate with light emanating from the very faces being depicted.

Near Gorky Park in Moscow, in Hamburg, Germany, at the Bellagio Hotel and Casino in Las Vegas, and in other locations around the world, music is calibrated to coincide with activity of huge water fountains illuminated dramatically with light. The choreographed combination of sound, light, and water can be quite mesmerizing.

Bellagio owner, Steve Wynn, conferred with designers of the Bellagio fountain in 1995, expressing his desire to create a fountain that "would be vibrantly kinetic and elating for visitors, while also expressing the romance of Bellagio." The fountains of Bellagio in Las Vegas are considered to be some of the most complex and impressive water fountains ever designed. They span over 1,000 feet in length with more than 1,000 water nozzles coordinated with 4,000 lights, which work in conjunction with specific musical patterns.

In its myriad applications, light is used to illuminate, entertain, or heal. The right type and design of lasers emit light in the form of photons that carry electrons to atoms at the sub-cellular level. In the next chapter, we will take a look at the basic principles behind laser physics.

Chapter 5

Basic laser physics

Nothing is faster than the speed of light.
To prove this to yourself, try opening the
refrigerator door before the light comes on.

Anonymous

Before we can discuss the laser light therapy that is the central purpose of this book, we need to understand the basic physics of laser therapy. Laser means Light Amplification by Stimulated Emission of Radiation.

Throughout the nineteenth century, scientists experimented with and theorized about electricity and magnetism; they already knew that flowing electricity generates a magnetic field. However, they had difficulty imagining a type of energy that required no medium to flow through; subsequent experiments were conducted that left no doubt.

British scientist, Michael Faraday, suggested there might be a link between electromagnetism and light. A fellow British scientist, James Clerk Maxwell, who was more a mathematician, predicted the discovery of wave radiation that traveled at the same speed as light within an electromagnetic field. Although he had no experimental proof, he theorized that light is electromagnetic.

Ten years later, Heinrich Rudolf Hertz, a German scientist, devised experiments that proved Maxwell's hypothesis about the nature of light. He succeeded in generating invisible radio waves; as a result, technology progressed swiftly. Subsequent experiments by Hertz showed that a medium such as air was not necessary for energy to flow between metal objects. Laser light, unlike sound, could travel through a vacuum as well.

In 1896, Italian inventor Gugleilmo Marconi patented his "wireless telegraph" device that used radio waves to transmit messages through "empty space." In 1901, his wireless signals spanned the Atlantic Ocean!

Albert Einstein, who, quite possibly was the most intelligent person who ever lived, first explained the photoelectric effect in papers published when he was just twenty-six in 1905. He proposed that light energy was transmitted in small amounts that he called "quanta," which would later be renamed "photons." His theories and ideas were so far ahead of his time that even now the most intelligent scientists alive are still discovering their value.

It was not until May 16, 1960, forty-three years after Einstein described the photoelectric effect, Theodore Maiman, an American research scientist at the Hughes Laboratory in Malibu, California, first theorized how lasers work that he developed the first laser—a ruby laser. The actual term 'laser' originated about three years earlier by Gordon Gould at the University of Columbia. Two physicists, Charles H. Townes and Arthur Schawlow, were the first to patent a laser and publish their findings in scientific journals.

Laser light differs from ordinary light in four ways:

1. It can carry information.

2. It is more directional.

3 It is monochromatic.

4 It is coherent.

You see, unlike normal light, which scatters and cannot carry information, laser light is coherent; that is, its waves run parallel and carry information, therefore it is much more valuable for therapeutic benefits.

The visible light red beam laser has been in commercial use since 1968. Many different lasers are in use today, for surgery, cutting metal, determining distance, projecting holographic images, and entertainment lighting. You've seen them at work in stores where a laser scans bar codes on your goods. You might have a printer with your computer, a pointer for use in lecturing, or a CD player, all equipped with lasers.

Pain results from trauma and/or cellular disruption, malfunction, or inferior cell function; normalizing the atoms that make up the cells promotes healing and minimizes pain. Wherever there is acute or chronic pain or inflammation, low level laser therapy can benefit. The QLaser System puts electrons back at the atomic pre-cell level and subsequently affects the entire body. Users have reported success treating arthritis, (the QLaser System received over-the-counter clearance for osteoarthritis of the hand in 2009), carpal tunnel syndrome, tennis elbow, whiplash, headaches (including migraines), back and shoulder pain, burns, cuts, sprains, cold sores, sinusitis, age spots, and diabetes. Treating Carpel tunnel and shoulder pain with low level lasers has received FDA clearance for prescription use.

CHAPTER 6

ENERGY MEDICINE

Health is not a condition
of matter, but of mind.

Mary Baker Eddy

Energy medicine deals with two types of energy fields: that which can be measured scientifically and that which has not yet been measured. The first is known as veritable energies: mechanical vibrations like sound, and electromagnetic forces, such as visible light, magnetism, and laser beams. They use measurable wavelengths and frequencies to treat patients.

Veritable or measurable energy medicine has been used to diagnose such as EKG, EEG, CAT Scan, and MRI. And it is also used to treat diseases: cardiac pacemakers, radiation therapy, ultraviolet light for psoriasis, laser keratoplasty, and others.

Used for centuries, people have experienced some relief of pain when static magnets are applied over a painful area of the body. Pulsating electromagnetic therapy has been used for the past forty years to treat osteoarthritis, migraine headaches, MS, and certain sleep disorders. Sound energy therapy acts on the basis that sound frequencies resonate with specific organs of the body for health and support. Music can help reduce pain and anxiety (some dental patients who wear headphones and listen to music during treatments could verify the effectiveness of this therapy).

On the flip side of measurable energy medicine are putative energy fields or biofields, which contend that human beings are infused with a subtle energy (electrons) that flows throughout the body. The difference between veritable and putative is that the latter has not been measured by conventional methods Techniques are being developed to measure the flow of electrons, but scientists still have trouble with something they can not see and are as elusive as the movement of electrons. Therapists, who practice this form of energy medicine often found in other cultures (China, Japan, and India), claim they can not only work with this subtle energy, but also they can see it (aura) and use it effectively to change the health and well-being of their patients. Auras were seen in the mid-1940s with the development of Kirlian photography in Russia and more recently documented in the United States with the development of bioliminal photography.

ELECTROMAGNETIC THERAPY

While it sounds like modern medicine, the roots of electromagnetic therapy reach all the way back to ancient Greece, Rome, and China. Of course, electricity had not been discovered, but the basic concepts of magnetism and energy were studied then.

With the discovery of electricity came the promotion of electromagnetic treatments with machines as early as the mid-1800s. Most of those devices were proven ineffective and even life-threatening, but some technologies have found a permanent place in modern medicine.

Albert Abrams, MD, is on record in the late 1800s with the first known use of frequency therapy with the development of several devices that he claimed could detect the frequencies of diseased tissue and heal the energy imbalances underlying the diseased tissue.

Since then, many devices have been created claiming to treat man's ailments, but the FDA has only cleared a few such devises, and because of the many unfounded claims has increased its efforts to control claims that are not backed by research. This will take a long time, because research measuring electrons is difficult to prove, according to today's research protocol. Science has, however, established that electrical and magnetic energy exists in the human body. Doctors use electrical energy to restart the heart after heart attacks or to promote bone growth.

Electromagnetic therapy, which includes electricity, microwaves, radio waves, infrared waves, and electronically-generated magnetic fields, uses energy to diagnose or treat disease. It is not the same as light therapy.

Such uses as the EEG, EKG, and other electronic devices have been medically approved to diagnose nervous system and heart problems, and to treat pain by interfering with nerve conduction of pain impulses.

As we stated before, when the body's energy fields lose electrons and go out of balance, disease and illness occurs. By applying electromagnetic energy through electric devices, practitioners can restore some of the energy balances in the body.

Therapists who utilize electromagnetic therapy can successfully treat a wide variety of ailments, from asthma and arthritis to cancer and spinal cord injuries. Some practitioners make claims that the scientific community cannot corroborate, and so certain electromagnetic therapy treatments receive little serious support in the medical and scientific fields. The problems with skin-induced devices to restore electrons back to the trillions of cells is skin application does not go very deep. It cannot reach all atoms of all cells at deep levels in the body.

Light therapy, also an example of measured energy medicine, employs lasers, colors, and monochromatic lights. We will go into more detail on this particular form of measurable energy medicine in subsequent chapters.

Energy medicine practitioners believe that illness is the result of disturbances of these subtle energies. Asian practitioners thousands of years ago held that the flow and balance of life energies are necessary for maintaining health; they used herbal medicine, acupuncture, acupressure, and other techniques to correct these imbalances in the body.

Reiki, Qi gong, healing touch, and intercessory prayer are some examples of putative energy medicine. Energy medicine is gaining popularity in America and has attracted the attention of academic medical centers for research and investigation. Medicine is being forced to accept that energy not only plays a role in illness; it also plays a major role in staying well and in the quality of life. Maintaining one's energy determines homeostasis, and when the body is in balance (homeostasis), there is no illness. Remember this author's definition of energy is movement of electrons.

Our bodies are just energy. When you die, if you choose to be cremated, 99 percent of your body mass goes up as energy in the form of heat; the remaining 1 percent is still energy in the form of charged minerals.

Long before that, however, there is the potential of extending life by treating common ailments with the use of properly designed and properly constructed low level lasers. Properly designed low level lasers deliver electrons back to the atoms that make up cells, that make up molecules, that make up tissue, that make up organs, that make up systems, which make up the body. In the next chapter, we will discuss the benefits of this alternative treatment, which is growing in acceptance and popularity and is an alternative to expensive, drug-based western medicine.

Chapter 7

Let There Be Light – Laser Light!

Energy and persistence
conquer all things.

Benjamin Franklin

If you are old enough, you may remember seeing science fiction comic books that used lasers to zap the enemy. It's not unusual that ideas so noted and seemingly far-fetched have become realities. We are more familiar with the military's laser-guided missiles and LASIK, a procedure that uses a laser to correct refractive errors, than we are with low level or "cold" laser that is a form of healing light that replenishes lost electrons at the cellular level due to aging, illness, elective and necessary surgery and injury.

Benefits of Low Level Laser Therapy

- Low level laser therapy is non-invasive.

- There are no known negative side effects.

- This therapy enhances cellular uptake of nutrition.

- It is an effective therapy for most conditions or injuries to the musculoskeletal system (back pain, arthritis, carpal tunnel syndrome).

- It can provide healing effects for wounds normally considered non-healing, as with diabetics ulcers.

- It is effective for dental and facial-related conditions, such as TMJ, neuropathies, gum infections, and bone loss.

- It supports the body's immune system.

- It helps to increase protein synthesis within the cells.

- It does not damage the skin.

- Low level laser therapy reduces or eliminates acute and chronic pain.

- It increases mobility and function.

- It promotes faster healing.

Low level lasers that produce less than one Mw (milliwatts) of power with an unfocused beam have been registered with the FDA to be 100 percent safe. In *Universal Healer*, this type of low level laser is termed "healing light" and works at the atomic level of the cell to restore lost electrons (energy), which helps the body heal injuries and reverse sickness and disease.

Our bodies are composed of cells; one human cell is so small that you would need an incredibly high-powered microscope to see it. Each human cell is made up of much smaller sub-atomic particles that are so tiny that it is difficult for the average person to even imagine their existence.

The health of our cells depends on energy. If they are exposed to excessive energy, they will be fatally damaged, and the body will die. On the other hand, if the cells receive insufficient energy, they will weaken, and the body will become sick or diseased.

To be healthy, the body's cells need exactly the right kind and amount of energy. Every time you get injured or become sick, the energy flow to your cells is disrupted. Until the proper type and amount of energy is restored, you will remain sick or injured.

That's the beauty of the low level laser. It re-energizes the cells in your body with just the right kind and proper amount of healing energy.

A low level laser is approximately the size of a cordless phone, is rechargeable, and is easy to use. Today, a growing number of doctors are using low level lasers to heal their patients; the specialty using them the most is sports medicine. The reason is quite easy to understand; these doctors must get their patients better and back on the playing field as quickly as possible. Every day that a professional athlete remains injured or out of play for health reasons, it can cost the sports organization millions of dollars. The player's team has a very high financial incentive to get the smartest doctors possible; often those are the doctors who know about alternative healing practices, such as the use of low level lasers.

The exciting news now is that you don't actually need to go to a doctor to get low level laser therapy. If you so desire, you can buy one of the devices and use it on yourself. The best ones come with simple, easy-to-use instructions and can be used by almost anyone with average intelligence.

After studying lasers for years, I have been fortunate to have invented some of the best low level lasers in the world. I speak from direct experience as an inventor, from personal use, and from testimonials and understanding that low level lasers put electrons back at the atomic level therefore can help almost every health problem experienced by both humans and animals.

If you hold a low level laser device against your skin and turn it on, you will be able to see the laser light, but you will not be able to feel its effects – oh, maybe a slight sensation of warmth – that's all. Laser light is as gentle as the kiss of a butterfly, but from a healing perspective, it is more effective than drugs and many times replaces surgery.

The problem of trying to explain the healing powers of low level laser therapy is that, because it works on so many different problems, people start to think it's too good to be true. But it is true! Just think about putting the electron back at the atomic level, and it won't seem like such a miracle.

As indicated earlier, all injury and illness creates an interruption of energy to human cells. The body will never recover until the proper type and amount of energy is restored to these cells. But once that energy is restored, the body can recover from almost anything.

Properly used, low level lasers can restore the correct energy flow to every cell in your body.

More than 2,500 studies have been conducted worldwide; they have shown that low level lasers:

- Reduce pain by stimulating cells to produce their own endorphins, a natural pain killer

- Promote faster healing by stimulating cells to increase the production of two major healing enzymes by as much as 75 percent

- Reduce inflammation by as much as 75 percent

- Increase bone repair speed

- Relax muscles and muscle spasms

- Decrease swelling

- Enhance the production of nitric oxide the cell-to-cell communicator by 400 to 900 percent.

- Enhance the immune system by increasing the number of "killer" cells by 400 percent to 900 percent, and most importantly

- Re-energize cell membranes to allow transport of essential nutrients across cell walls (nutrients will not cross a depolarized, injured, or sick cell membrane, thus slowing healing), allowing a healthy new cell to grow.

NO MORE ACUPUNCTURE NEEDLES!

Needle acupuncture has been around for thousands of years, and many eastern cultures have touted its effectiveness. Regardless of what the acupuncture doctor says, getting stuck with a needle still hurts and arouses fear in most people. And forget about trying to do traditional needle acupuncture yourself! Even if you could locate the correct points, assuming they are located on an accessible part of the body, it would still require an extreme amount of skill to do it properly. This problem has been solved with the correct type and power of low level laser.

After years of research, I devised a small handheld diode laser that can stimulate the acupuncture points with a beam of light tuned to a specific frequency that benefits the human body, and which you can easily use yourself. This laser device can concentrate laser light at the acupuncture points or at a broad expanse of multiple acupuncture sites on the body, depending upon which laser model is being used.

Many books on the market illustrate the traditional Chinese acupuncture points. *Low Level Laser Application Guide* includes a section that shows the points that can be activated with low level laser light as a substitute for needles. The procedure for stimulating acupuncture points with laser treatment is very easy.

Following a user-friendly guide, anyone can learn to use a safe low level laser instrument that emits the correct amount of energy for their own laser acupuncture therapy. One simply aims it at the area of the acupuncture point and switches on the laser for approximately a minute. The comforting therapeutic and preventive medical effects that result often amaze practitioners who administer low level laser therapy on their clients, as well as those who use it on themselves.

Chinese and other Asian healers readily accept the use of low level laser therapy on acupuncture points. Their minds are open to new technologies, which can be combined with ancient healing methods. Joining acupuncture points with laser light is the ultimate example of the benefits to be derived from the integration of modalities and technologies from different traditions. In Japan, for instance, cold or soft lasers have been approved for treatment since 1987 and are widely used today.

Romeo Quini, MD, a family practice physician, is a good example of a traditional medical doctor embracing the new technology of low level laser therapy. Dr. Quini received his initial medical training in the Philippines and served two residencies in general and thoracic surgery in Chicago. He learned classical acupuncture and herbology from a traditional Chinese doctor and has used acupuncture in his medical practice since the early 1970s.

Ten years later, he began using low level laser light to replace the needles. His results for patients have been superb, but let's hear it directly from Dr. Quini, as he wrote in March 2003:

> I have been using Dr. Larry Lytle's low intensity laser in my medical practice for nearly two years. I utilize the principles of acupuncture points. They work in a fantastic manner for most medical ailments! As a physician, I have used low level laser therapy for many medical conditions with very good results. The conditions include: trauma (hematomas resolve quickly, and sprains and strains find almost instant relief); arthritic pains (my patients achieve fast relief when some cases cannot be helped by conventional medications); and postoperative pain. As a surgeon, I have used low intensity lasers for control of many types of pain. Many of my patients do not need pain medications because of my application of post-operative low level laser therapy. They also recover faster."

Dr. Quini's clinical research tested about fifty diabetics under a set protocol with the QLaser System. The results have been outstanding! He did not expect it to be like this. From all results, lowering of sugar levels has been almost consistent on his trial cases.

A 2010 Russian study reports using multiply diode low level laser therapy on approximately sixty diabetic patients from the age of three to seventy-three called applied magneto-infrared-laser therapy (MILT) with very positive results. Blood sugar levels dropped by 50 to 200 mg/100ml in 98 percent of the subjects after each low level laser session. Subjects reported that pain syndrome complications, cardiomyopathy, nephropathy, diabetic foot ulcers, reduction of obesity, and erectile dysfunction nearly completely disappeared. Treatment with MILT during the three-to-six-week period resulted in completed recovery of diabetic foot ulcers with full soft tissue regeneration and restoration of local blood circulation. The Russian doctors stated that regardless of the type of diabetes, when the patients observed all recommendations blood sugar levels normalized at between 60-90 mg/100ml and the patients did not need any more insulin or hypoglycemic tablets. More than 60 percent returned to drinking and eating sweets in normal amounts, while the rest observed diet restrictions

At the six-year follow-up, neither a recurrence of pathological hyperglycemia nor another apparent manifestation of diabetes mellitus has been reported in any of the patients treated by the method of bioresonance information laser therapy.

The doctors who did the study—Dr. B. Shkalar Head of Pain Unit Kaplan Hospital; Dr. C. Daniel, head of orthopedic unit, Hillel Yaffe Medical Center; Prof. S. Edelstein, Weizmann Institute of Science; Dr. W. Simon, Internal Medicine Specialist, Rambam Medical Center; Multidisciplinary Medical Center, Tel Aviv; and Prof. H., head of orthopedic unit, Assaf Harofeh Medical Center—stated: "The first most important conclusion made during this clinical-experimental study is that even in advanced cases of diabetes mellitus, the pancreas retains its ability to restore the functional possibilities of its tissues as well as their regeneration, specifically the insulin-producing ß-cells of the Islets of Langerhans. Otherwise, without the functional restoration and structural regeneration of these islet cells, it would have been impossible to bring down the blood glucose level to normal values without the use of any exogenous hypoglycemic medications. It should be well noted that the common thought, that it is impossible for the pancreas to restore its function and morphology in cases of diabetes mellitus, has definitely come to an end in the history of this disease and man- kind. Secondly, it has been ascertained from this study that the quantum energy of laser rays is capable of stimulating and causing the regeneration of pancreatic tissues, including the ß-cells of the Islets of Langerhans, even in advanced disease states."

LOW LEVEL LASER SYSTEMS

Low level lasers come in many forms, shapes, and powers. The operating source of the laser is a laser diode—a chip, not unlike diodes used in other areas of electronics. An analogy can be made between transportation and low level lasers. A horse, bicycle, small car, big car, train, bus, boat, single-engine plane, or super fast jet are all modes of transportation. The consumer knows which mode he needs and what to buy, but it is not that way with lasers.

Even though lasers have been around for forty or more years, many consumers may have never heard about the benefits of low level laser therapy, and some of those that have may consider "a laser is a laser is a laser." But not all low level lasers are created equal. Depending on size and power, lasers have different uses, so it is very important to know how to use them.

As an example of misinformation, some advertisements, salespersons, and even some doctors say that a laser pointer or an LED light will work for various health benefits. Laser pointers are small, very low-powered single diode lasers; their intended purpose is for use in lecturing, teaching, surveying, and at home, not for healing.

LED means light-emitting diode. LEDs are similar to the red, blue or green lights on the dash of your car. For healing, LEDs have some benefit in reducing surface inflammation but cannot compare to true lasers that emit coherent light and carry information. LEDs are not coherent light and cannot carry information.

These instruments are inexpensive to make and cheap to buy. While all light works at least to some extent, this type of laser pointer is really a waste of money; it is considered a "toy" when it comes to treating and healing the body and mind.

Some manufacturers believe that you need only stimulating lasers; others, only resonating lasers. Which is correct?

To Resonate or to Stimulate: That is the Question

In order for you to understand how low level lasers can treat Type II diabetes, we must first define resonate and stimulate. Resonate is defined as vibrate or to get in harmony; stimulate means to invigorate, awaken.

To determine if a low level laser is resonating or stimulating depends on the amount of energy the laser emits as measured in milliwatts (Mw) and in joules. Generally, the laser industry and the FDA consider anything under one watt or 1000 Mw as a low level laser. Resonating low level lasers are under 5 Mw and stimulating low level lasers are between 5 Mw and 500 Mw.

The rule for using low level lasers is to:

✧ resonate organs, glands, and bellies of muscles; and

✧ stimulate nerves, cartilage, tendons, joints, and bones.

Resonating low level lasers are battery-driven multiple diode lasers that produce less than 5 Mw of energy and harmonize with the body. Lasers powered by 110 or 220 volt AC (alternating current) have too much electromagnetic contamination running down the electric line and are not as efficient as DC battery-driven lasers for producing resonating energy.

Cellular research reported in Dr. Bruce Lipton's book, *Biology of Belief,* takes a new look at the role of our body's cells, particularly the cell membrane. Lipton states that our cells control our body, and the cell membrane is the brain of our cells. All cells generate light in the infrared wavelength called biophotons. When these biophotons join together, they produce a soliton wave that flows through the body on the liquid crystalline matrix of the cells. They carry important information and are the "brains" of the body.

The beauty of the QLaser is that it is a resonating multiple-diode laser with delivery of patented soliton waves, just like the body's cells do. They deliver energy in the form of electrons back to the cell membrane and normalize the messenger system. Another benefit of multiple diode low lever lasers is the various wavelengths, and since one wavelength will not do it all, you get a "shotgun" approach, a "cover the waterfront" approach.

A stimulating low level laser, on the other hand, is one that emits from 5 Mw to 500 Mw of energy. Stimulating lasers are usually single-diode lasers; that is, they contain only one wavelength. While the wavelength may vary, the most common stimulating lasers are in the red or near-infrared range.

Lasers are named according to their wavelength, as measured in nanometers (Nm). A laser that produces a red light ranges from 635 Nm to 670 Nm. Infrared lasers—those you cannot see—ranges from 780 Nm to 905 Nm.

Single wavelength lasers cannot produce a soliton wave, and therefore the depth of penetration is limited, depending on the wavelength. Red or visible light lasers do not penetrate as deeply as infrared or invisible lasers. Red light lasers are used more for acupuncture or surface treatments, while infrared is better for deeper penetration of joints, tendons, ligaments, nerves, and bones.

More powerful is not better and does not insure deeper penetration, which is better accomplished by combining laser diodes to produce the soliton wave.

All this information considered, are low level lasers safe? In the next chapter, we will look at the issue of safety and give assurances that they can be used safely, even in the home.

Chapter 8

Low Level Laser Therapy – Safety

For safety reasons, every electronic device carries a warning label about the danger of possible injury; however, most low level lasers are not really dangerous. Consider those used by cashiers to read bar code on product labels. They are not dangerous for two reasons: (1) the power of the scanner beam is minimal and considered a Class I device (the scanner will not damage the eye), and (2) the natural act of blinking offers further protection, even if one looks directly into the laser light.

Nevertheless, because laser light can be concentrated into a narrow beam, which focuses on a small spot, such as a handheld laser pointer, it is much brighter than conventional light, and therefore shining a laser into the eye is not recommended.

Quickly glancing at the sun does not injure the eyes, but a long stare directly at the sun over a long period of time can damage the retina. In the same way, low-power lasers will not damage the eyes, but if someone deliberately stared at the laser light for a period of time, it could be dangerous.

Despite their acknowledgment of the safety of low level lasers, the FDA warns parents and school officials of the potential danger of hand-held laser pointers in the classroom. The FDA, alarmed about the possibility of eye damage to children from such pointers, wants people to know that the products are generally safe when used as intended, but sometimes children and adults use them inappropriately.

As the FDA points out, it is not the laser light that is dangerous; it is the misuse of the device by a foolish adult or curious child that could be harmful. When laser lights are employed for their intended purposes, they carry no hazard. As stated, the FDA has issued safety guidelines for manufacturers and operators of laser light shows, and the agency's officials state publicly, "When used safely, low level lasers are not dangerous."

There is another important distinction between the common consumer lasers, such as those used to scan bar codes, and industrial lasers used in factories to fabricate metal. Lasers, in fact, can be powerful enough to cut metal. The cutting edge of such industrial lasers begins with a wide beam that is focused by bending the light rays symmetrically, using a short-focal-length lens, which concentrates the light at an intense focal spot. The laser beam's power can be extremely high. The light that pulses from a commercial/industrial cutting laser almost instantly eats into and melts the metal at the focal point. If you were to look at this type of laser without safety glasses, your eyes would be permanently damaged in a fraction of a second.

The low level lasers described in this book are not powerful enough to do any cutting. Regardless of how long they are used, they will not create damage. Low level laser therapy works at the cellular level to restore the cells to health. In fact, low level laser instruments are sometimes referred to as "healing lights"!

According to Sanford Simon, professor of biochemistry and pathology at the Stony Brook Health Sciences Center, School of Medicine, Department of Pathology, in 2000, they completed the first phase of evaluating a set of low energy laser devised. "These results strongly suggest that the lasers are truly safe for human use and do not induce cytotoxicity when employed at the maximum recommended exposure period."

The data used, although not requested to be specifically designed for applications to federal agencies for use with human volunteers, was "fully consistent with the type of results frequently sought by such agencies as evidence of safety and tolerance when the devices are used as recommended."

LASER SAFETY CATEGORIES

The intensity of light beams produced by lasers depends on the design and the pump that injects energy into the core. There are four FDA categories based on the intensity of laser light output and the potential risk to the eye. Class 1 represents the least risk, and as the power gets progressively higher in Class 2, Class 3A and 3B, and Class 4 lasers, the risk for eye damage increases.

A Class 1 laser, described by the FDA as a "non-significant risk device," is considered safe based upon current medical knowledge. This Class 1 category includes all lasers or laser systems, which cannot emit levels of optical radiation above exposure limits, tolerated by the eye under any exposure conditions inherent in the design of the laser product.

A Class 2 laser or laser system must emit a visible laser beam. Because of its brightness, its laser light will be too dazzling to stare into for extended periods. Momentary viewing is not considered hazardous, but intentional extended viewing is considered hazardous. No known skin exposure hazard or fire hazard exists. Lasers used to read bar codes in stores fall into this safety category.

Class 3A includes most laser pointers on the market today and emits a visible blue, green, or red light. These lasers are considered more hazardous to the eyes than Class 1 or 2 lasers, because they are focused. They should not be looked at directly at close range for extended periods of time. Because the eye blinks when it is exposed to a bright light, a temporary exposure to the eye will not cause permanent eye damage.

Class 3B lasers are usually infrared, which means they are not within the visible spectrum of the eye and cannot be seen; therefore, the blinking effect is not activated, and this class of laser could cause damage to the eye if misused. Do not look directly into this laser, unless you are wearing protective eyeglasses.

A Class 4 laser or laser system is any device that exceeds the output limits. These lasers may be a visual hazard, and protective glasses are required when using them. Cutting lasers belong in this safety category. Very stringent control measures are mandated by the FDA for use of Class 4 lasers.

FDA APPROVAL

Lasers are being used throughout the world. Medical specialists can join the American Society for Laser Medicine and Surgery, the Academy of Laser Dentistry, the International Society for Lasers in Dentistry, the North American Association for Laser Therapy, and the World Association for Laser Therapy.

In 1996, Congress instructed the FDA to study low level laser devices and their efficacy for treating disease. Since then, the FDA and the National Institutes of Health have been in the process of carrying out several such studies. Since the FDA requires the study of the effect of low level laser therapy on each disease (there are hundreds of classifications of diseases), it will take generations for them to complete the studies to show the many benefits of low level laser therapy.

In 2004, the FDA approved them for treatment of myofascial pain of the shoulder and for carpal tunnel syndrome. Low level laser therapy practitioners hope that the FDA will soon change their protocol and conduct general studies of the effect of low level lasers at the cellular level, where they actually do their work. Since the body is composed of cells, it makes sense to study low level laser therapy effectiveness on cells, rather than on the many diseases.

As of 2009, the FDA cleared the QLaser System for treating the symptoms of osteoarthritis of the hand. [See letter of approval in the beginning of this book.]

In short, the FDA has determined that exposure to low level laser light is safe for human beings. Its experience with other laser devices approved for medical use has given them a more open mind toward low level lasers. Recognizing that the risk to a patient's health posed by low level lasers is very little to none at all, the FDA has shown uncommon restraint in its oversight authority.

The FDA has already issued approvals for low level laser therapy devices and does not appear to have any objection to issuing more in the future. Some companies have made such advances in the laser therapy field that they have won FDA approval, while others are awaiting approval. The U. S. government is using low level lasers in VA hospitals, and the military is conducting research into use of low level light therapy.

Given the fact that the FDA has already approved many medical laser procedures, it seems likely that the use of low level laser devices for the treatment of nearly every type of dysfunction will gain approval in the near future. Such approval will allow any person to use this safe and inexpensive low level laser therapy to the relief of his or her osteoarthritis and diabetes. Since there is very little risk to the self-treating, the FDA will probably approve low level lasers for home use by all Americans.

Also, as noted earlier, the FDA has approved over-the-counter sales of low level lasers for the treatment of osteoarthritis of the hand. Similar FDA approval for treatment of Type II diabetes should express the same conditions and terms as the earlier approval.

CHAPTER 9

TYPE II DIABETES CLINICAL STUDIES

Clinical Research Proves the Effectiveness of Low Level
Laser Therapy for Type II Diabetes

The FDA not only requires low level lasers to be approved for safety, it also requires clinical studies to demonstrate the effectiveness of these lasers before any pre-market claims can be made by the manufacturer. The general consensus among clinicians using low level laser therapy for conditions having an inflammatory component (such as Type II diabetes) is that significant benefits could be accumulated by those patients treated with this type of laser.[1]

PLACEBO CONTROLLED STUDY USING THE QLASER SYSTEM

The purpose of this clinical study was to determine the effectiveness and feasibility of over-the-counter (OTC) use of the QLaser System made up of the Q1000 low level laser device and the 660 nm FlashProbe, manufactured by Tri-Tech Manufacturing Inc. in providing adjunctive use in reducing and maintaining or reducing HbA1C blood levels at a normal to low-risk level for those diagnosed with Type II diabetes. Treatment was administered by an individual in his or her own home.

Clinical Study

This QLaser System clinical study was planned to be submitted to the FDA for clearance or approval; therefore the study followed accepted protocol for FDA submission. The study was a placebo-controlled, randomized, double-blind, parallel group study design, meaning that the user did not know if he or she was using a real laser or a placebo (fake) laser. It was carried out over a six-week period in Turkey on eight-eight patients suffering from Type II diabetes. Forty-four patients were treated with real lasers, and forty-four were treated with fake lasers. All subjects, whether assigned the treatment or placebo group, received the same treatment protocol.

Inclusion Criteria

To be included in the study, all subjects had to satisfy each of the following inclusion criteria and could not have any of the exclusion criteria. The subjects had to be diagnosed with Type II diabetes mellitus (formerly called NIDDM, Type II or adult-onset), which is characterized by insulin resistance in peripheral tissue and an insulin secretory defect of the beta cell, and is diagnosed and verified through HbA1c analysis. In this study, HbA1c blood levels were considered normal if the subject had readings of less than 6.5 to 7. If HbA1c levels were above 7.2, the subject qualified for this study. Inclusion criteria were based on the diagnosis of diabetes using criteria from the following organizations:

- Report of the Expert Committee on the Diagnosis and Classification of Diabetes Mellitus. Diabetes Care 1997; 20:1183-97.

- National Diabetes Data Group. Diabetes in America. Bethesda, Md.: National Institutes of Health, National Institute of Diabetes and Digestive and Kidney Diseases, 1995; NIH publication no. 95-1468.

- American Diabetic Association (ADA) criteria for Type II diabetes

Other eligibility requirements were:

- Willing and able to abstain from consuming new over-the-counter or prescription medication(s) for Type II diabetes-related symptoms, commencing sixty hours immediately prior to administration of the first treatment using the study devices, and up until the time of his or her final visit to the test site six weeks later.

- Able and willing to use only authorized prescribed medication (study rescue medication and patient prescribed medication) during the course of the study for Type II diabetes symptoms and agree to follow the directions for use.

- Willing and able to abstain from partaking in any existing or new treatments (non-pharmacological) for Type II diabetes, commencing sixty hours prior to administration of the first study treatment, and up to the time of completion of his or her participation in the study about six weeks later.

- Be at least 18 years of age

- The following exceptions applied and were left to the discretion of the doctor conducting the study:

Usually most Type II DM cases are elderly men or women, so it may be difficult to cancel their medication(s) for six weeks. Not using any medication(s) may be unethical for placebo cases. No medication for six weeks may be seen unacceptable by the ethics committee.

EXCLUSION CRITERIA

The following subjects were excluded from participation in the study for the following reasons:

- Current use of any one or more of the following medications: narcotics, opiates, morphine, steroids, Vitamin C (it may affect the HbA1c levels)

- Type I Diabetes Mellitus

- History of severe or multiple allergies

- Treatment with any other investigational drug or adjunctive therapy for Type II diabetes within three months of trial entry

- Progressive fatal disease

- History of drug or alcohol abuse

- History of significant cardiovascular (>NYHA stage II-IV), respiratory, gastrointestinal, hepatic (ALAT >2.5 times the normal reference range), renal (creatinine > 1.2 mg/dl), neurological, psychiatric, and/or hematological disease

- Blood donation within the last thirty days

- Lack of compliance or other similar reason that, the investigator believes, precludes satisfactory participation in the study

- Developmental disability or cognitive impairment that would make it difficult to partake in the study and record the necessary measurements

- Significant psychological disorder for which hospitalization has become necessary

- Pregnancy or lactation

- Participation as a subject in any type of study or research during the prior ninety days.

- Using insulin's parenteral forms for treatment Type II DM.

QLASER SYSTEM

The QLaser System is composed of two separate lasers: The Q1000 and the FlashProbe. The Q1000ng is powered by a high capacity lithium-ion rechargeable battery. The battery is placed inside the device and is <u>not</u> removable by the user. To charge the battery, the user plugs the device into either 110v or 220v electrical outlet with the supplied power supply. During charging, the unit will not operate in its regular manner. All internal devices are powered, but the software does not allow the user to interact with the unit. The battery charger is specially designed to operate with lithium-ion batteries and closely monitors charge current as well as maximum allowed voltage. In addition, the battery is supplied from the battery manufacturer with a safety charge/discharge circuitry to prevent overcharging or over-discharging of the battery. The redundant nature of this approach creates a safe power delivery system.

The Q1000ng is fitted with a 24-pin multi-use external connector to connect the instrument to the charger or to connect other external compatible devices.

How to Use the Q1000ng Laser for Type II Diabetes

The following written directions were given to each participant, and they were told to follow these directions. The subjects were told to apply the Q1000ng as follows on days 1, 3, 5, 8, 11, 15, and 18.

STEP 1: Apply the Q1000ng to proprioceptive points 1, 2, and 3, as shown in the picture diagrams. First, turn on the Q1000ng by pressing the ON/OFF button one time. Then immediately apply the laser to the left proprioceptive point just in front of the left ear over the TMJ until the unit beeps one time— approximately one minute. (For those reading this book who are using an older model of the Q1000, press the mode button one time to mode one and apply for approximately one minute, which unusually equals about six to eight deep breaths, or follow the directions in your *Low Level Laser Application Guide)*

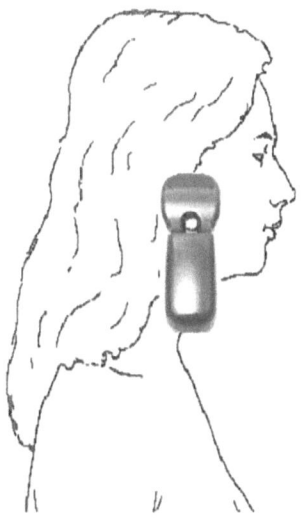

Q1000ng applied to left proprioception point in front of ear

Without delay, immediately move the Q1000ng laser and apply to the left proprioceptive point under the angle of the jaw with the laser pointed upwards at a 45-degree angle until the unit beeps two times—approximately one minute. (For those reading this book who are using an older model of the Q1000, press the mode button one time to mode one and apply for approximately one minute which unusually equals about six to eight deep breaths, or follow the directions in your *Low Level Laser Application Guide)*

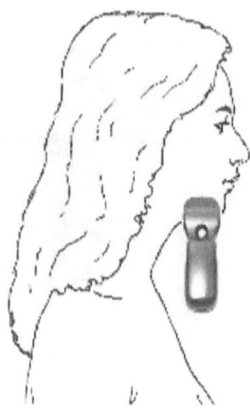

Q1000ng applied to left proprioception point at the angle of the jaw

Without delay, immediately move the laser and apply to the left proprioceptive point two finger widths below the collar bone and three finger widths in from the armpit until the unit beeps three times—approximately one minute. (For those reading this book who are using an older model of the Q1000, press the mode button one time to mode one and apply for approximately one minute which unusually equals about six to eight deep breaths, or follow the directions in your *Low Level Laser Application Guide)*

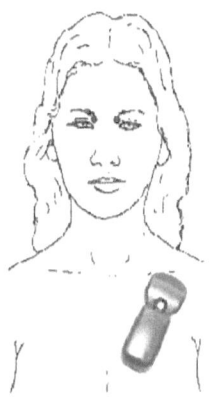

Q1000ng applied to left proprioception point below collar bone

STEP 2: Without delay, immediately turn the Q1000ng back on by pushing the ON/OFF button one time and repeat STEP 1, but apply the Q1000ng to three proprioceptive points on the right side of the body.

STEP 3: Without delay, immediately turn the Q1000ng back on by pushing the ON/OFF button one time and immediately move the laser and apply over the neck below the Adams apple over the "V" where the collar bones meet for one cycle—three beeps or until the laser shuts off. (For those reading this book who are using an older model of the Q1000, press the mode button one time to mode one, and apply for approximately one minute which unusually equals about six to eight deep breaths, or follow the directions in your *Low Level Laser Application Guide)*

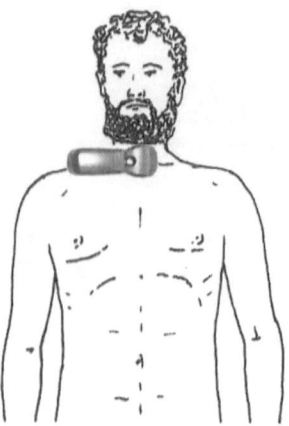

Q1000ng applied to the thyroid area

STEP 4: Without delay, immediately turn the Q1000ng back on by pushing the ON/OFF button one time and immediately move the laser and apply over the left kidney (best placement to reach the pancreas) in the small of the back—approximately one-hand width above the belt and one-hand width to the left of the spine for three cycles—three beeps or until the laser shuts off. (For those reading this book who are using an older model of the Q1000, press the mode button one time to mode one and apply for approximately one minute which unusually equals about six to eight deep breaths, or follow the directions in your *Low Level Laser Application Guide*)

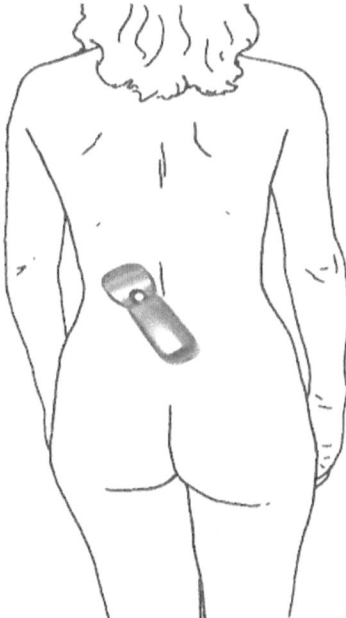

Q1000ng applied to the pancreas over the left kidney area

STEP 5: Prepare for 660ng FlashProbe application. As soon as you finish the treatment with the Q1000ng Laser, immediately begin the treatment with the 660ng FlashProbe, as indicated below. With the Q1000ng turned OFF, plug the cord of the 660ng FlashProbe into the end of the Q1000ng and without delay; turn the Q1000ng back on by pushing the ON/OFF button one time. Immediately apply the 660ng FlashProbe to a spot one hand width below and in line with the navel until the unit beeps one time—approximately one minute

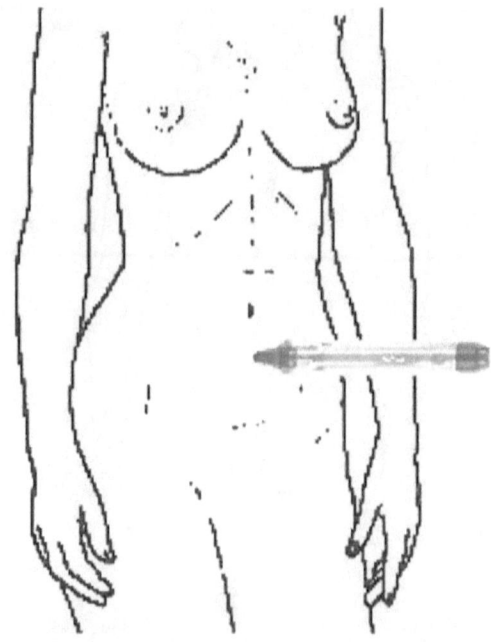

STEP 6: Immediately move the laser and apply the 660ng FlashProbe to the spot at the extreme end of the inner crease of the elbow. To locate the point, bend the arm tightly and place the probe tip at the extreme edge of the elbow crease, relax the arm, and apply until the Q1000ng for two beeps—approximately one more minute.

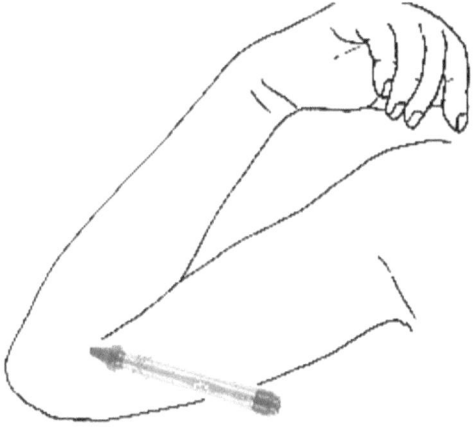

660 FlashProbe applied to acupoints at crease of elbow

Treatment is now complete. Press the MODE button two times in rapid succession (double-click) to return the Q1000ng to Standby Mode. Now press the ON/OFF button one time to turn the unit off.

SUMMARY OF HOW THE QLASER SYSTEM WAS USED

The Q1000ng laser was used directly against the skin on proprioceptive points, as shown in the above pictures, three times on week one for one minute on Days 1, 3, and 5, then on week two it was used two times on Days 8, 15, and it was applied again the next week on Day 18. The final application was on Day 42 at which time the HbA1C blood test was made and recorded. All subjects followed the same treatment administration protocol, regardless of whether they were assigned to the treatment group or to the placebo group. The only difference was that for subjects in the treatment group, the actual laser device was used, while for subjects in the placebo group, a sham laser device employing an LED light was used. The Q1000 Laser was applied directly to the skin on the proprioceptive points for one minute each on Days 1, 3, 5, 8, 15 and 18.

RESULTS

As mentioned earlier, certain blood cells, called A1C cells, are used as a marker for Type II diabetes. Over a three-to-four-month period of time, A1C cells become glycolated; that is, they load down with sugar in people who cannot handle sugar. Sometimes this blood test is referred to as HbA1c. Hb refers to hemoglobin in the blood and the A1C is the blood cells tested.

The American Diabetes Association uses a 7 percent HbA1C, and the American Association of Clinical Endocrinologist recommends a maximum HbA1C of 6.5 percent. The results, as demonstrated by the HbA1c blood levels in this study of the treatment group over fake or placebo treatments, were clinically significant. Sixty-nine percent of the treatment group demonstrated a drop in HbA1C levels in just forty-two days. In reading the test results in another way, the treatment group started lowering HbA1C levels at the end of the first week and continued the trend to lower the test scores at the end of six weeks. Consult the results chart on the following page.

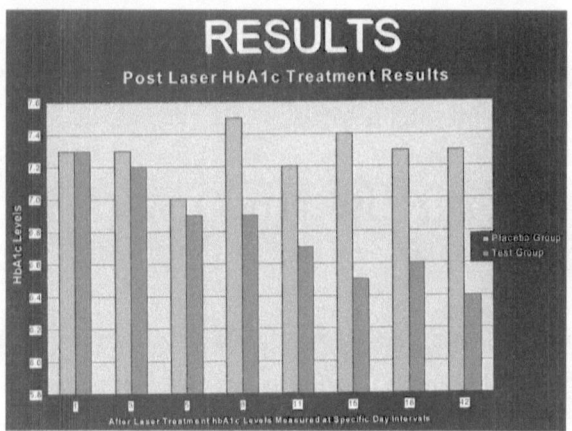

Authors Stratton, Adler, and Neil state that for every 1 percent decrease in A1C, it significantly lowers the risk of micro-vascular and macro-vascular complications. Vascular complications lead to other disorders, such as heart attack, brain vessel leakage, and stroke.

RUSSIAN STUDY ON TYPE 1 AND TYPE II DIABETES

A 2010 Russian study reports a 98 percent success in controlling both Type I and Type II diabetes when using multiple-diode low level laser therapy. The study was conducted on approximately sixty diabetic patients from the age of three to seventy-three. The low level lasers were accompanied by what they called applied magneto-infrared-laser therapy (MILT) to enhance penetration. (As previously stated the QLaser System study relied on the Soliton wave, a patented diode technique to provide penetration). The diodes used in the Russian were similar to the diodes used in the QLaser System's double-blind, placebo-controlled study, but the Russian study did not mention the number of joules delivered or length of treatment time. They reported that blood sugar dropped by 50 to 200 mg/100ml in 98 percent of the subjects.

In the preliminary survey, the subjects reported various conditions such as: pain syndrome complications, cardiomyopathy, nephropathy, diabetic foot ulcers, obesity, and erectile dysfunction. In the final survey of those treated by low laser therapy, these conditions nearly completely disappeared. Treatment with what the Russian doctors called MILT during the three-to-six-week period resulted in completed recovery of diabetic foot ulcers with full soft tissue regeneration and restoration of local blood circulation. Furthermore, the Russian doctors stated that regardless of the type of diabetes, when the patients observed all recommendations blood sugar levels normalized at between 60-90 mg/100ml, and the patients did not need any more insulin or hypoglycemic tablets. An amazing 60 percent of the subjects returned to drinking and eating sweets in normal amounts after low level laser treatment.

At the follow-up visits, neither a recurrence of pathological hyperglycemia nor another apparent manifestation of diabetes mellitus has been reported in any of the patients treated by this method of bioresonance information laser therapy. It appears that both Type I and Type II diabetes was **cured.**

The doctors who did the study—Dr. B. Shkalar Head of Pain Unit Kaplan Hospital; Dr. C. Daniel, head of orthopedic unit, Hillel Yaffe Medical Center; Prof. S. Edelstein, Weizmann Institute of Science; Dr. W. Simon, Internal Medicine Specialist; Rambam Medical Center, Multidisciplinary

Medical Center, Tel Aviv; and Prof. H., head of orthopedic unit, Assaf Harofeh Medical Center—stated: "The first most important conclusion made during this clinical-experimental study is that even in advanced cases of diabetes mellitus, the pancreas retains its ability to restore the functional possibilities of its tissues as well as their regeneration, specifically the insulin-producing ß-cells of the Islets of Langerhans. Otherwise, without the functional restoration and structural regeneration of these islet cells, it would have been impossible to bring down the blood glucose level to normal values without the use of any exogenous hypoglycemic medications. It should be well noted that the common thought, *that it is impossible for the pancreas to restore its function and morphology in case of diabetes mellitus, has definitely come to an end in the history of this disease and man- kind.* (Emphasis added) Secondly, it has been ascertained from this study that the quantum energy of laser rays is capable of stimulating and causing the regeneration of pancreatic tissues, including the ß-cells of the Islets of Langerhans, even in advanced disease states."

Russian study results show 98 percent returned to normal blood sugar

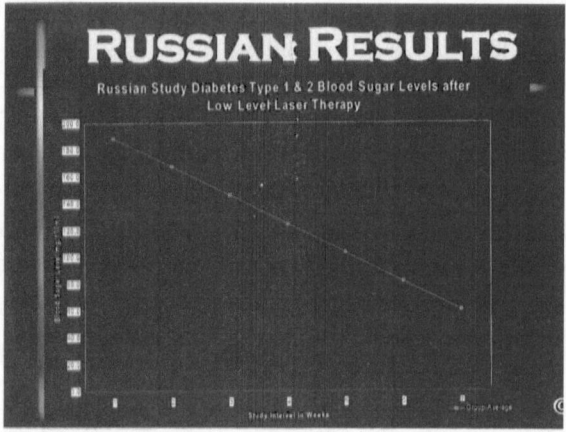

This author adds that if a pancreas can heal from low level laser therapy, so can other organs such as the heart, the liver, the kidney, the stomach, and, in fact, the entire body.

FDA APPROVAL

The FDA was discussed earlier, but I want to emphasize that the FDA does not actually approve low level lasers or any other over-the counter devices, for that matter. In fact, one has to wonder why the FDA even controls non-significant risk devices such as low level lasers. It seems the marketplace should decide the fate of non-significant risk low level lasers—not the government. However, at this time, the FDA gives authorization to market devices for their intended purpose. The public usually refers to this process as approval. The QLaser System was given FDA clearance to market it for over-the-counter sale for osteoarthritis of the hand January 30, 2009.

The QLaser System works at the atomic level by replacing lost electrons on the trillions of human cells. Current FDA protocol does not think at the atomic level. They want laser devices studied strictly from the disease symptom standpoint. With that in mind, the QLaser system has an application pending with the FDA to seek clearance of the QLaser System for Type II diabetes by reducing HbA1c and blood glucose levels.

N-of-1 (One) Studies

N-of-1 trials are a means of conducting research on an individual patient with the added opportunity to use patient-generated outcome measures. Patients act as their own control and receive all treatments under comparison, more than once, in a random sequence. While N-of-1 trial methodology is reasonably well specified, they remain under-exploited, and little is known about the process aspects of conducting such trials or the experiences and views of those who participate in them. N-of-1 trials rely on cooperation between individual clinicians and patients. Each reader can participate in an N-of-1 study by keeping their records and reporting them to your distributor on the N-of-1 template as shown below.

N of 1 Study Submission Form			
Participant	Age:		Sex:
	Race:		Location:
Condition – please describe as accurately as possible			
Purpose of Study	Pain Reduction		Inflammation Reduction
	Stiffness/Mobility (describe)		Other (describe)
Pre-Treatment Score – rate from 1 (lowest pain, inflammation, etc.) to 10 (highest pain, inflammation, etc.)			

Equipment Used In Treatment. Note: if you used previous versions of equipment please mark the current equivalent.	Q10	Q1000	660 Flash Probe	808 Flash Probe

Describe the Treatment Process. I.e., how many minutes per treatment, how many treatments per week, how many total weeks the treatment took.

Post-Treatment Score – rate from 1 (lowest pain, inflammation, etc.) to 10 (highest pain, inflammation, etc.)

Satisfaction With Treatment	Very Dissatisfied	Somewhat Dissatisfied	Neutral	Somewhat Satisfied	Very Satisfied

Additional Related Information

Date Study Was Conducted	Participant Initials

Following are several N-of-1 trials. Some studies are on diabetes and others are on other conditions. Please submit your special findings to your laser distributor.

CASE STUDY
Di
Caroline Barton
London, England

(While this case was not officially diagnosed as osteoarthritis of the hand, the symptoms were the same)

I had a very painful area in the base of my thumb on the inside of my left palm, from years of pressing heavily on my walking stick. Some days, I can hardly move the thumb. The area between the wrist and thumb base is swollen and red with inflammation. Up until using the multi-diode, multi-wavelength, multi-frequency low level laser, the only help for the pain was a sports ice pack.

I found to my amazement that after only one session of holding this special laser over the sore area, it resulted in greatly noticeable reduction of pain, allowed movement of the thumb joint, and even the skin color became light pink from having been red blotchy.

Whilst I am obliged to continue using my walking stick, which exacerbates the problem, daily use of my laser could be my salvation!

CASE STUDY
Sports Injuries
Doug Phillips
Rapid City, South Dakota

My name is Doug Phillips, past president of the SD Racquetball Association, and competitive open level player. I am forty-five years old and have played multiple sports all my life. In 1990, I was diagnosed as having ankylosing spondylitis (arthritis) fusing of the spine and hips, and had a 'titanium cage' implanted in my back in 1999. In 1990, I also ruptured the Anterior Cruciate Ligament (ACL) in my right knee, and was told by two different orthopedic surgeons that I would need a total knee replacement.

I didn't have the surgery, and continued, as best I could, an active lifestyle while fighting the pain with a combination of anti-inflammatory drugs and pain killers prescribed by my doctor—neither of which worked very well at all. The knee was still inflamed and caused a great deal of pain.

While at the YMCA for a lunch time racquetball session in September of 2001, Dr. Larry Lytle allowed me to use his low level laser on my right knee. I lasered the knee for about three minutes before and after playing that day. The results were amazing. I was able to play a full hour and half of racquetball, and go back to work without any pain or inflammation!

I continued to use the laser approximately three times per week (during our lunch time racquetball sessions) for the next three weeks, and continue to be amazed by what low level laser therapy has done for me. My right knee is pretty much back to normal, with no pain and no inflammation! Thank you, Dr. Lytle, for introducing me to this incredible equipment!

CASE STUDY
Osteoarthritis &
Type II Diabetes

Ben Gieringer

I have my own personal lasers and have been lasering the front area and on acupoints for my diabetes. This helped, and my blood sugar scores went down from about 260 to 190.

Since talking to you, I followed through on the two things you told me—to use the laser on my lower back for the pancreas and to also laser my thyroid. My results have been dramatic, and my blood sugar scores went down to 120 and have remained there. I have also stopped taking my 15mg of Prednisone that I have been taking for two years.

Dr. Lytle, thank you for sharing your knowledge and thoughts with me.

CASE STUDY
Chronic Neck Pain, Lower Back Pain & Pet
Injuries

Tamara Shearer, DVM

Our hospital's first experience with the low level laser was with me. I have suffered from chronic neck pain that was so intense it could make me cry. After one treatment (laser) my pain was gone and it has been in remission for one and a half months now. All of my staff that has had painful necks, lower backs, and feet is now comfortable.

The goal of my investment was to improve the comfort of pets that suffer from pain or to expedite healing of disease conditions. Just today, we treated seven patients with low level laser. Three of the most dramatic improvements include Theo, Maggie, and Nike. Theo is an eight-year-old cat with a cruciate injury of three months' duration. Before his knee surgery, he received three laser treatments, and his lameness was resolved. His owner cancelled his surgery.

Maggie is a thirteen-year-old beagle that had lower back disc problems and bilateral cruciate surgery in the past. She would moan and groan when trying to lie down. After her first treatment, she climbed on the kitchen counter and ate the cat food. Nike is a five-year-old Schnauzer with severe back pain. After his first treatment, he is pain-free.

CASE STUDY
Myofascial Pain Syndrome in the Neck
Gur A, Sarac AJ, Cevik R, Altindag O, Sarac S

In this study taken in 2004, a prospective, double-blind, randomized, and controlled trial was conducted with patients who suffered with chronic myofascial pain syndrome in the neck. Sixty patients were included in the study to evaluate the effects of low level laser therapy on quality of life. The therapy continued daily for two weeks, except weekends. All patients were evaluated with respect to pain at rest, pain at movement, number of trigger points, and other clinical criteria.

In the active laser group, statistically significant improvements were detected in all outcome measures compared with baseline; while, in the placebo laser group, significant improvements were detected in only pain score at rest at one week after the end of treatment.

The score for self-assessed improvement of pain was significantly different between the active and placebo laser groups (63 percent vs. 19 percent, respectively). This study revealed that short-period application of low level laser therapy is effective in pain relief and in the improvement of functional ability and quality of life in patients with this painful condition.

CASE STUDY
Chronic Myofascial Pain in the Neck
Gur A, Sarac AJ, Cevik R, Altindag O, Sarac S

A double-blind, randomized, and controlled trial was conducted to determine the efficacy of low level laser therapy in the management of chronic myofascial pain in the neck. The score for self-assessed improvement of pain was significantly different between the active and placebo laser groups (63 percent vs. 19 percent, respectively). This study revealed that the short-period application of low level laser therapy is effective in pain relief, in the improvement of functional ability, and qualify of life in patients suffering this painful condition.

CASE STUDY
Sports & Traffic Accident Injuries
Z. Simunovic, MD, A. Ivankovich, MD, A Depolo,
MD

The main objective of this study was to assess the efficacy of low level laser therapy on wound healing in rabbits and humans. A randomized controlled study in rabbits initially evaluated the effects of laser irradiation on the healing of surgical wounds. The application of low level laser therapy to human tissues is comparable to animal tissues of similar physiological structure.

After surgical therapy for injuries involving the ankle and knee bilaterally, Achilles tendon, shoulder, wrist, or interphalangeal joints of the hands unilaterally, low level laser therapy was used in seventy-four patients for eighteen days. The presence of redness, heat, pain, swelling, and loss of function were assessed.

Wound healing was significantly accelerated (25 percent to 35 percent in the group of patients treated with low level laser therapy. Pain relief and functional recovery of patients treated with low level laser therapy were significantly improved, compared to results of the untreated patients.

In addition to accelerated wound healing, the main advantages of low level laser therapy of postoperative sports- and traffic-related injuries are reduced exposure to side effects of drugs, significantly accelerated functional recovery, earlier return to work, training and sports competition, with cost benefit compared to control patients.

CASE STUDY
Tennis & Golfer's Elbow
Z. Simunovic, MD, T. Trobonjaca

In a two-center, double-blind, placebo-controlled clinical study, 324 patients with unilateral medial or lateral epicondylitis (tennis and golfer's elbow) were treated with low level laser therapy. Total pain relief was obtained in 85 percent of the acute cases and 66 percent of the chronic cases. A combination of trigger points and scanning was more effective than trigger points alone, and trigger points alone was more effective than scanning alone. One of the centers had slightly less powerful lasers, and the outcome was a bit lower, although the dosage was the same in both centers.

CHAPTER 10

HOW TO SELECT A LOW LEVEL LASER

Several questions should be answered before the consumer buys a low level laser to treat Type II diabetes or other conditions. Here are some of the more important questions:

- *Should I buy a single-diode or a multiple-diode laser?* A multiple-diode laser system is best, because one wavelength will not do everything.

- *What are the benefits of each laser?* Multiple-diode low-powered lasers resonate, while single-diode, higher-powered lasers stimulate. Both are needed to treat Type II diabetes.

- *Is more power better? What power of laser should I buy?* More power is not better for organs, glands, and releasing bellies of muscles, but more power is better for nerves, bones, ligaments, and tendons; therefore, it is best to buy a laser system, not a single laser.

- *How is the amount of laser energy measured? Is more energy better?* In low level lasers, dose is measured in joules and is determined by the power of the laser, how long it is used, and size of the laser beam. More does not insure deeper penetration or better results.

- *Should I buy an AC (alternating current 110 or 220 volt) or a DC (direct current, battery-powered) laser?* AC is okay for stimulating, but it is not good for resonating. DC computer-regulated battery-powered lasers are best for resonating.

- *If I buy a DC-powered unit, what power is best? Should I buy one that is computer controlled?* Less than 5 Mw is best for resonating organs, glands, and bellies of muscles, but it is important that the battery output is regulated by an internal computer. If not, as the battery bleeds down, the power will fluctuate, the body will set up impedance, and the results will not be as good.

- *Should I buy a laser with multiple frequency capability?* Frequency capability is important. Some lasers come with built-in frequencies, and others allow the operator to program in their own frequencies. Our entire universe is a vibrating conglomerate of frequencies. The big question is which frequencies are best for which disorder. At this time in low level laser therapy, not enough is known about canceling and constructive frequency, but buying a laser with the capability of adding frequencies later when we know more is good.

- *Should price be the main determining factor in buying a laser? What price should I expect to pay?* Being an intelligent buyer is always important, but price should not be the major criterion for choosing a laser; function is. When buying a multiple-diode laser system, you can expect to pay from $3,800 to $8,000.

- *How important is service and warranty?* Service and warranty are very important, <u>more important than price</u>. Buy your laser from a company that has been in business for a long time and that offers readily available service and stands behind their product with a good service, as well as a satisfaction warranty. Beware of foreign-made lasers; you may not be able to get them repaired in the United States.

- *Don't be fooled by LEDs.* There are many light devices on the market that may look like lasers and are pawned off as lasers, but really are just LEDs—that is, light-emitting diodes or colored lights similar to those on the dash of your car reminding you that a door is not closed. While all light may have some benefit, be sure you are getting a real laser.

- Remember laser companies come and go, and service and warranties are worthless if the company goes out of business. Study and know the company, before you buy a laser.

Chapter 11

Low Level Laser Benefits More N-of-1 Studies

Many patients with symptomatic Type II diabetes have been treated with various types of low level laser therapy. To date, several double-blind studies, N-of-1 clinical studies, and more than 2,500 research reports have been published demonstrating the positive clinical effects low level laser therapy.

The following is a collection of studies evaluating the use of low level laser therapy for adjunctive use in reducing and maintaining HbA1c blood levels at a normal to low risk level for those diagnosed with Type II Diabetes Mellitus.

Clinical Study

The following is a report of a clinical study completed on the clinical efficacy of low level laser therapy for Type II Diabetes Mellitus in Escondido, California, by Dr. Romeo Quini.

Dr. Quini started clinical trials on forty adult-onset diabetic patients using low level laser acupoint therapy as the main treatment modality. Two times a week, Quini applied a multiple diode 5mW low level laser programmed with twenty-nine different proprietary frequencies (mode 3 of the Q1000) directly over the pancreas and applied a 660nm – 30mW laser probe to acupuncture points located on the body, known as proprioceptive points.

The patients maintain their medications and diet as prescribed by their physicians. Supplements are encouraged, and, if desired, recommendations are given. Prior to commencing the clinical trial, patients were asked how their current medications and diet maintain their blood glucose levels at a normal to low risk level. Eighty percent of the patients that participated in the clinical study reported that they were unable to lower their blood sugar levels to normal despite medications and diet prescribed by physicians.

After one month of Low Level Laser Therapy, 100 percent of the patients showed no increase in HbA1c levels. Ninety-five percent of the patients, both on oral and insulin therapies or both, showed a gradual lowering of HbA1c levels. Seventy-five percent of the patients were able to reduce medications as HbA1c levels became lower. Two percent of the patients studied became hypoglycemic and stopped taking their medications altogether, but maintained laser therapy. Five percent of the patients studied had episodes of mild HbA1c level elevations, to be followed by gradual lowering. Even with small elevations, they did not get higher than the former high levels. In other words, the levels were still lower than the original HbA1c levels tested at the beginning of the trial.

Fifty percent of the patients with other symptoms, in addition to Type II DM, such as blurred vision, double vision, weakness, cramps, abdominal and leg pains, shortness of breath and others, reported the symptoms improved or disappeared after the second or third low level laser therapy.

CLINICAL STUDY

The following is a report of a clinical study completed by Dr. Larry Lytle over a sixty-day period on Robert Rumph. At the time of the clinical study, Rumph was seventy-six years old and had been treating his Type II diabetes for twenty-five years with various oral drugs and diet. Rumph used low level laser therapy twice a week on the proprioceptive points indicated in this protocol.

Rumph's blood sugar levels were over 250, on an average of 80 percent. Prior to commencing this clinical study, Rumph was facing a required insulin program. Rumph's blood sugar level tested at 254 on the first day of the clinical study. After one week of the clinical study, Rumph's blood sugar level tested at 220. After two weeks of the clinical study, Rumph's blood sugar level tested at 180. After another two weeks of the clinical study, Rumph's blood sugar level tested at 153. After sixty days of the clinical study, Rumph's blood sugar level tested at 121, a dramatic decrease from 254.

Rumph reported he had been having a terrible time controlling his diabetes. He said: "I was using the cold laser (low level laser) treatments in front (going through the stomach) under the first rib and was getting nothing done—no results, and couldn't figure out what might be wrong with the instrument. I went to Gillette to see my—Dr. Billy Wilkerson. She said that the front is the spleen. 'To get to the pancreas, you need to laser on the back (left side) below the first rib.' I've been using the laser on my pancreas now for a week. When I started, my blood sugar was 254. She said, 'I'll let you go for another three or four months to see if you can get your blood sugar down, but if you can't, you'll have to go on insulin.'

"We came home, and I started using the laser on my back, and my blood sugar started dropping about 20 points every day! It went from 245 to 220, down to 210, down to 180. On January 1, it was 184, and then it dropped to 161 and then again to 153, then to 136, and then to 133. Today, it was 96 on one machine and 121 on the other. That's down from 154 in a week's time!

"I test my blood with two different instruments—a One Touch and a Dex machine. The One Touch is supposed to be accurate, but you have to handle the glucose strip with your fingers, which can possibly contaminate the strip.

Interview with Robert Rumph on January 6, 2003

Dr. Lytle: How long did you use the Q1000?

Robert: I just used it one three-minute cycle per day on Mode 3 on the lower left side of my back beneath the first and second ribs. My daughters have been buying me everything they can thing of to help with my diabetes

– none of that garbage worked! I'm going to stop using this other garbage and will continue to use the laser.

Dr. Lytle: What I might suggest is for you to stop using the laser for a week or ten days and see if your blood sugar goes back up.

Robert: Oh, I know it would.

Dr. Lytle: You could really be a big help to a lot of people with diabetes if you could set some type of standard for how many times per week you have to use the laser to keep your blood sugar under control.

Robert: I think that two times per week are all I'm going to need to use it.

Dr. Lytle: Yea, I don't think you're going to need to use it every day to keep your sugar level down. I would ask you to help us out by stopping using it for a week and document the results. If it goes back up, then use the laser twice a week and record the results.

Robert: I want to run it down a little lower. (blood sugar)

Dr. Lytle: Anything under 120 is pretty normal. Have you changed anything on your diet?

Robert: No, I haven't really changed anything, but have pretty much the same diet as always.

Case Study on Type II Diabetes
Ben Gierenger

The following is a report of a clinical study completed by Dr. Larry Lytle over a sixty-day period on Ben Gierenger. At the time of the clinical study, Gierenger was fifty years old and had been treating his Type II diabetes for ten years with Prednisone and diet. Gierenger used low level laser therapy twice a week on the proprioceptive points indicated in this protocol and the 660 probe for acupoints. Gierenger's blood sugar levels were first recorded at 260 at the beginning of the clinical study. After applying the laser three times a week on the proprioceptive points with the low level laser and the acupoints with the 660 probe, Gierenger tested his blood sugar level at 120. Gierenger's blood sugar levels remained at an average of 120 with continued laser therapy for the next thirty days. During this time he discontinued taking Prednisone but maintained laser therapy. I have my own personal lasers and have been lasering the front area (with the Q1000) and using the 660 (Enhancer) on acupoints for my diabetes. This helped and my blood sugar went down from about 260 to 190.

Since talking to you, I followed through on the two things you told me—to use the laser (Q1000) on my lower back for the pancreas and to also laser my thyroid. My results have been dramatic, and my blood sugar scores went down to 120 and have remained there. I have also stopped taking my 15mg of prednisone that I had been taking for two years. Dr. Lytle, thank you for sharing your knowledge and thoughts with me.

Case Study

The following is a report of a case study conducted by P. Weldy, an individual owner of the QLaser System, on a fifteen-year-old female diagnosed with Type I Diabetes Mellitus. The subject was taking twenty-two units of insulin per day. In two treatments using low level laser therapy on the acupoint and proprioceptive points, she has reduced insulin requirements to two units per day.

Case Study

The following is a report of a case study conducted by T. Oba, an individual owner of the QLaser System, on a fifty-eight-year-old woman diagnosed with Type II Diabetes Mellitus and kidney deficiency.

At the onset of using the QLaser System, the patient was told that her kidneys were only functioning at 9 percent, and she tested 220 for blood sugar levels. She was told that if her kidney deficiency rate could not elevate to 15 percent, she would have to commence kidney dialysis. After forty-five days of treatment with the QLaser System on proprioception points, the patient reported her kidney deficiency was up to 36 percent and her blood sugar levels had dropped to 110. She was told she could reduce the amount of medication to treat her Type II Diabetes Mellitus.

Lasers Used to Preserve Eyesight in Diabetic Patients

In a recent multi-center study, funded by the National Institute of Health's National Eye Institute, laser therapy is now considered to be more effective than corticosteroids in the long-term treatment of diabetic macular edema (DME). "Many of the investigators, including myself, were surprised by the results," said Dr. David Brown, ophthalmologist and retina specialist at The Methodist Hospital in Houston and local principal investigator. "We're continually researching new treatments, but sometimes the tried and true methods are still the best course. These findings substantiate the importance of laser treatment in the management of diabetic macular edema." In addition to being more effective, laser therapy has considerably fewer side effects. This is important news for the 40 to 45 percent of 18 million Americans diagnosed with diabetes who have vision problems, such as diabetic macular edema, a condition that occurs when the center part of the eye's retina (macula) swells, often leading to blindness.

Competence in Wound Healing

The following images show the healing of diabetic gangrene in a male patient, sixty years of age, with Type II diabetes. The third toe of his left foot developed gangrene. Conventional therapy did not lead to healing of the tissue, and an amputation was performed. After the amputation, new gangrene occurred. Laser therapy, administered in a clinic in Austria, treated the toe over an eight-week period. The therapy was successful and led to complete healing.

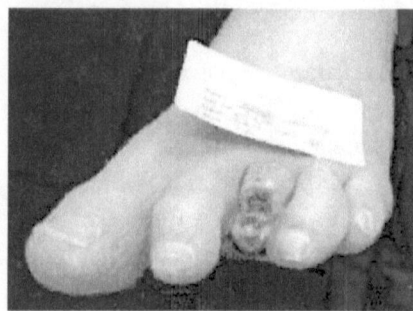
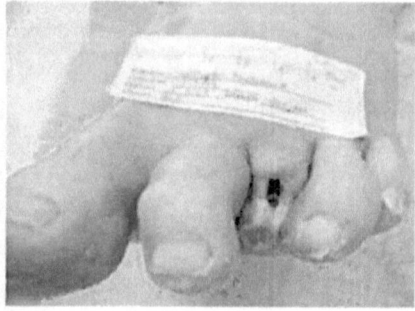

Before laser therapy   After 2 weeks laser therapy

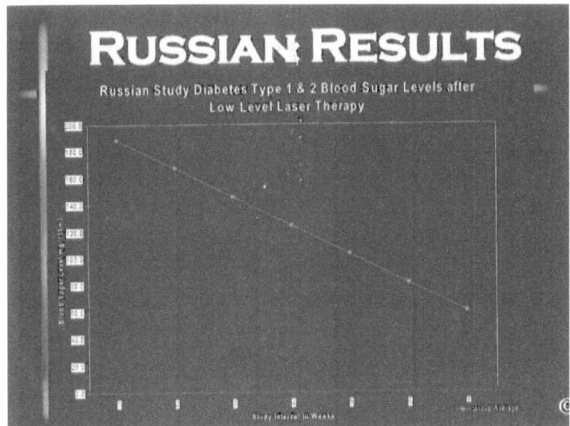

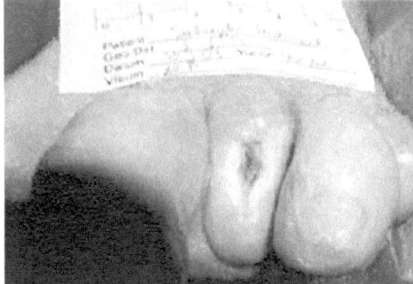
After 4 weeks laser therapy

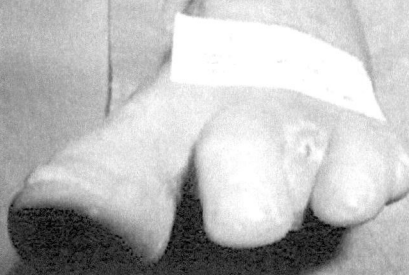
After 8 weeks laser therapy

N of 1 Study Submission Form

Participant	Age:		Sex:		
	Race:		Location:		
Condition – please describe as accurately as possible					
Purpose of Study	Pain Reduction		Inflammation Reduction		
	Stiffness/Mobility (describe)		Other (describe)		
Pre-Treatment Score – rate from 1 (lowest pain, inflammation, etc.) to 10 (highest pain, inflammation, etc.)					
Equipment Used In Treatment. Note: if you used previous versions of equipment please mark the current equivalent.	Q10	Q1000	660 Flash Probe	808 Flash Probe	
Describe the Treatment Process. I.e., how many minutes per treatment, how many treatments per week, how many total weeks the treatment took.					
Post-Treatment Score – rate from 1 (lowest pain, inflammation, etc.) to 10 (highest pain, inflammation, etc.)					
Satisfaction With Treatment	Very Dissatisfied	Somewhat Dissatisfied	Neutral	Somewhat Satisfied	Very Satisfied
Additional Related Information					
Date Study Was Conducted			Participant Initials		

TESTIMONIAL - MIGRAINE HEADACHES

My wife had migraine headaches for thirty years. Being a chiropractor, we had tried every sort of natural approach we could find to beat the headaches. Nevertheless, she had to eat every two hours to keep her blood sugar stable, and needed to take four ibuprofen capsules every night before bed in order to keep the headache at bay. After starting the laser and receiving the bite tabs, within two to three weeks, she became free of migraine headaches and does not need to eat every two hours or take ibuprofen anymore. We used Mode 2 for the headache, Mode 1 for the muscular tension at the occipital, and Mode 3 for the pancreas. I'm sure the bite tabs helped quite a lot as well. —Steven Hecht, Washington, DC

Testimonial—Bone Healing & Diabetes

My father at age nine was one of three given insulin injections after the team of Banting and Best discovered its beneficial use in lowering blood sugar in previously untreatable diabetics.

I was eight years old when I first started receiving insulin injections for diabetes. I remember the anxiety I felt when harsh realities were told as lessons in teaching control of my new "condition." My aunt had a leg amputated. My uncle was blind, due to this silent destroyer of body parts—diabetes. I was grateful when home blood testing became available; before that, urine testing was the only measure of blood sugar control. The results in urine testing were always several hours off. Today, the real "miracle" is the healing light laser. I moved into a new home, and within a year, I had three falls, breaking the three small toes on my right foot. I found after the bones were healed, my foot would not hold me up. I would fall to the right. The doctor said it was neuropathy, and nothing could be done for this condition. I felt my old anxieties flooding over my mind and into my stomach.

I saw an article about the healing light laser treating neuropathy. I sucked my breath in; my eyes opened wide; and hope began. I talked my husband into going to the seminar with me. The information I heard gave me new excitement to be alive again, and although it sounded too good to be true, it fit logically. If sick cells could be repaired, they could have renewed life. The seminar was in January 2008; this is March 2008. The laser has proven its miraculous healing power. I now have feeling in the three previously numb toes. I am happy to be wearing my sandal-foot high heels again, to walk without worry of falling; especially to banish the anxieties of the complications of my "condition."

When we attended the seminar, my husband faced the possibility of having prostate surgery. He used the low level light laser, as Dr. Lytle demonstrated at the seminar. It has been five weeks. On my husband's last visit to his surgeon, he was told his prostate was greatly improved, and he would not need surgery.

These are the first miracles we have experienced, and we have had the laser for three months. I am presently using the laser on our Pekinese. Our vet said her kidneys are not functioning well. The last blood test she had showed poor kidney values. I am using the laser on Mode 3, three or four times a week over her kidney areas. I expect the next blood tests will show improvement.

It is remarkable to see how an instrument so simple to use can send such tremendous healing benefits to the body and mind. I am very grateful for Dr. Larry Lytle through his genius and compassion for humanity he created the Healing Light Laser without limit on healing power. —Coni Mathews, Rancho Mirage, CA

Chapter 12

Universal Healing – Looking to the Future

In health, there is freedom.
Health is the first of all liberties.

Henri Frederic Amiel

With the potential to help virtually every health problem experienced by humans, I firmly believe that low level laser therapy will become the medicine of the future, but more than that, for many people who have already discovered the benefits that low level laser therapy imparts, it is the medicine of today.

Of course, there are and will be skeptics. "If it works so well on so many different problems; it sounds too good to be true." But it is true! All injury and illness creates an interruption of energy to the cells of the human body. The body will never recover until the proper amount and type of energy is restored to these cells.

Once that energy is restored, however, the body can recover from almost anything! Properly used, low level lasers can restore the correct energy flow to every cell in your body.

This information just might help relieve you of any disease and possibly save your life and the lives of your loved ones.

For some people, a book like *Universal Healer* marks the beginning of an entirely new life…pain-free and full of energy. For others, it can make a difference between living a healthy life compared to a low-energy life of sickness, disease, and disability. For still others, it helps those who live with enormous pain every day of their lives to exchange it for a life that is 100 percent pain-free.

Even if you are not sick, injured, or in pain, you should still learn as much as you can about low level laser therapy. After all, almost no one lives a lifetime without some sickness or injury. Wouldn't it be nice to know that, if you become sick or injured, you will know where to go to find some sort of answer to your problems?

NEW USES OF LOW LEVEL LASER THERAPY

The American medical culture rarely blazes new trails, but succeeds more often in perfecting treatments and medical instruments that doctors and researchers in other countries pioneer. LASIK eye surgery, first developed in Greece, followed the example of Soviet ophthalmologist, Dr. Svyataslov Fyodorov, and his development of radial keratotomy for the correction of myopia. In both cases, American ingenuity stepped up to the plate, and in both cases raised those procedures to the high standards of American medicine, so, too, we have researchers and physicians in other countries looking at new applications of low level laser therapy. In Colombia, biomedical researchers discovered that low level laser therapy can break up fat. Imagine what that would do to the diet industry in the United States! Talk about the Holy Grail!

Doctors in Turkey found that patients suffering from fibromyalgia responded well to low level laser therapy. The cause of this muscular and skeletal pain and fatigue disorder is still unknown; its sufferers experience terrible discomfort in their muscles, ligaments, and tendons. They "ache all over," and their muscles feel like they have been overstretched or overworked. After treating fibromyalgia patients with low level laser therapy, a Turkish physician observed: "Significant improvements were indicated in all clinical parameters (disease symptoms) in the laser group." These improvements included: reduced pain, reduced number of tenderness areas, less joint stiffness in the morning, more restful sleep, less muscle spasm, and less fatigue.

Near infrared light therapy, also known as low level laser therapy, is drawing a lot of attention from research clinicians around the world. For a number of years, various research centers in Japan, Britain, and the United States have been conducting clinical trials to measure the effectiveness of red and near infrared light over injuries and lesions. The results show that they contribute to healing and provide relief for both acute and chronic pain.

Many of these trials have proven to be very successful and clearly verify that light can have a positive effect on damaged cells. Continued research into the benefits of low level laser therapy surface regularly and bring great excitement to the very real reality of universal healing.

Chapter 13

Frequently Asked Questions

What is Type II diabetes?

Type II diabetes, once referred to as adult-onset or non-insulin-dependent diabetes, is a chronic condition that affects the body's metabolism of sugar (glucose), our primary source of fuel.

The pancreas of a Type II diabetic produces either an insufficient quantity of insulin, or the body does not recognize it or utilize it properly. This is known as insulin-resistance. Either situation prevents glucose from entering the body's cells, resulting in build-up of glucose in the blood, causing improper functioning of the cells, among other problems, such as dehydration, diabetic coma, and damage to many of the body's vital organs.

What causes Type II diabetes?

Our body's main source of energy of the cells is glucose, which is derived from two major sources: food that we eat and our liver. Digestion helps sugar to become absorbed into the bloodstream, and then into the cells with the help of insulin.

Normally, the pancreas secretes insulin into the bloodstream. As this vital hormone circulates, it serves as a catalyst, allowing sugar to enter the cells.

Insulin lowers the amount of sugar in the bloodstream, and as the blood sugar level drops, the pancreas cuts back its secretion of insulin.

Another vital organ is the liver, which stores glucose for times when your insulin level drops—such as when you have not eaten in awhile. During those times, the liver releases stored glucose to keep your glucose level within a normal range.

For Type II diabetic people, this whole process doesn't work correctly. Instead of sugar moving into their cells, it builds up in their bloodstream, and then the pancreas cannot manufacture enough insulin or their cells become resistant to the action of insulin. It seems that excess fat—especially abdominal fat—and inactivity are important factors to help explain it.

What are conventional treatments of Type II diabetes?

Conventional treatments of Type II diabetes include weight loss and weight control, dietary changes, increased exercise, insulin (oral or by injection), and diabetes medications.

What are the drawbacks to the conventional approach to treating Type II diabetes?

In our desire to fix things more quickly and to keep up with the trends in modern medicine, we are prone to rush to the latest "fix-it" remedy. However, this habit has its drawbacks, because:

- Newer drugs are no better and less effective than those that had been on the market for years, even decades.

- Newer drugs offer no greater safety; all anti-diabetes medications carry the potential to trigger side effects, some serious.

- Newer drugs are more expensive.

- When it is sometimes necessary to take more than one diabetes drug, doing so raises the risk of adverse side effects and increases costs.

Are there any natural or holistic treatments of Type II diabetes?

There are many alternative and holistic treatments of Type II diabetes, ranging from acupuncture and aromatherapy to herbs and dietary supplements to meditation and yoga. Maintaining proper dietary guidelines, as set forth by the patient's physician and nutritional specialist, is mandatory, particularly if obesity is present. Adhering to even a minimum amount of daily exercise can be effective in controlling blood sugar.

How does laser light differ from normal light?

Lasers are coherent wave lengths of light that travel in a straight beam until something absorbs them. Regular light is scattered, filling a space instead of traveling in a straight line like laser light. Laser light also differs in that it can carry information. These qualities make laser light much more valuable for therapeutic use.

Are low level lasers safe?

YES! Low level lasers have been used for many years (bar code checkouts, CD players, laser printers, and laser pointers). The FDA describes them as "non-significant risk devices." Moreover, the FDA says that "when low level lasers are used safely, they are not dangerous."

How do they work?

Pain arises from trauma and/or cellular disruption, malfunction, or less than optimal cellular function. Healing and pain relief come when the cells are normalized. Photons enable cells to perform optimally by stimulating them to initiate bio-chemical reactions, which produce enzymes and usable energy.

Have low level lasers been scientifically studied and their effectiveness proven?

Low level lasers have been used worldwide for more than thirty years. Over 2,500 studies have shown that low level lasers 1) reduce pain, 2) promote faster healing, 3) reduce inflammation, 4) increase bone repair speed, 5) relax muscles and muscle spasms, 6) decrease swelling, 7) enhance the immune system, and 8) re-energize cell membranes.

Where can low level laser therapy be used?

Low level laser therapy can be used any place where there is acute or chronic pain or inflammation, and it may be used effectively to treat any disease or disorder—Type II diabetes, arthritis, carpal tunnel syndrome, tennis elbow, whiplash, headaches, back and shoulder pain, burns, TMD/TMJ, cuts, sprains, colds and cold sores, sinusitis, and even age spots.

Why haven't I heard about low level lasers until now?

There are several reasons why low level laser therapy may be one of the best kept secrets in the world. Among them are: 1) mainstream medicine has not endorsed low level laser therapy as they have hotter, cutting types of lasers; 2) insurance companies are slow to accept and pay for low level laser therapy; 3) low lever lasers are a threat to the highly lucrative pharmaceutical companies and healthcare industry, because they work too well, do not need to be replaced, and do not require a doctor or other healthcare practitioner to administer the treatment; 4) unbiased research money is hard to come by; 5) absence of a low level laser manufacturing association to set standards and guidelines; and 6) hesitance on the part of mainstream media to release news on the success of low level lasers, largely due to the fact that it does not generate a flood of advertising dollars like they receive from pharmaceutical companies.

Where can I go to get low level laser treatment?

While there are many medical doctors, energy doctors, naturopathic doctors, dentists, chiropractors, osteopathic doctors, and other healthcare providers using low level lasers, there is no central list for you to consult. And, since low level lasers are completely safe, it is best, more convenient, and more economical for you to own your own laser equipment to treat your family and you in the comfort of your own home.

How much do low level lasers cost?

If you buy a single-diode low level laser, it can cost as little as $39 for an effective laser pointer, and up to $190 for a LED-only device. Computerized therapeutic multi-diode, multi-wavelength, multi-frequency low level lasers cost much more. Professional therapeutic lasers cost more than home-use lasers. Do your homework and study which laser is best for you, and do not let cost be the determining factor when buying a low level laser.

Where can I get more information about low level lasers?

There are two low level laser associations with websites that publish ongoing information: The World Association of Laser Therapy (WALT) at www.WALT.org, and the North American Association of Laser Therapy (NALT) at www.NALT.org.

Also, there are many websites owned by various companies, each promoting their low level laser products. While each company quotes its own choice of research to promote its products, there is still considerable unbiased information on low level lasers. When reading these sites, remember one laser, one wavelength will not do everything a combination of wavelengths will do.

The following references are good sources for more information on low level lasers:

1. Laser Therapy by Tuner and Hode

2. Healing Light by Dr. Larry Lytle

3. Healing Light DVD, a 16-hour series by Dr. Larry Lytle

4. Low Level Laser User's Manual by Dr. Larry Lytle

5. Test and Grow Healthy by Dr. Buddy Frumpker

6. The Rife Frequencies by Dr. Nina Silvers

7. Energy Transcendence by Dr. Larry Lytle

8. Universal Healer Book 1 Osteoarthritis – Dr. Larry Lytle

For a list of distributors of the low level laser system used in the QLaser System clinical Type II diabetes study discussed in this book, contact QLaser Solutions at www.Qlasersolutions.com.

Chapter Sources

Introduction

"Diabetes – Disabling Disease to Double by 2050"
Source: Center for Disease Control
www.cdc.gov/needphp/publications/aag/ddt.htm

"New US Diabetes Rate Up 90 Percent in Past Decade"
Reuters News Story, October 30, 2008
www.diabetes.org

Type 2 Diabetes
Chris Woolston
Consumer Health Interactive
www.ahealthyme.com

Diabetes Facts
www.peacefulmind.com/diabetes.htm

Chapter 1

"Diabetes – Disabling Disease to Double by 2050"
Source: Center for Disease Control
www.cdc.gov/needphp/publications/aag/ddt.htm

"Incidence of Diagnosed Diabetes among People Aged 20 Years or Older,
United States, 2007"

National Institutes of Health
http://diabetes.niddk.nih.gov/dm/pubs/statistics

National Diabetes Statistics, 2007
National Institutes of Health
http://diabetes.niddk.nih.gov/dm/pubs/statistics
"Direct & Indirect Costs of Diabetes in the United States: 2007"
American Diabetes Association
www.diabetes.org/diabetes-statistics/

"Complications of Diabetes in the United States"
National Diabetes Statistics 2007
http://diabetes.niddk.nih.gov/dm/pubs/statistics

Diabetes Guide
Source: WebMD
http://diabetes.webmd.com

Type 2 Diabetes
www.mayoclinic.com

"Stress of Dealing with Diabetes Linked to Depression"
John Gever, MedPage Today
June 17, 2008
Journal of the American Medical Association

"The Truth about Diabetes"
Walter Last
www.health-science-spirit.com/diabetestruth.htm

"Study puts a total on diabetes cost: $218 billion
Linda A. Johnson, AP Business Writer
www.yahoo.com

"Diabetes drug costs soaring, top $12B last year (2007)
Diabetes News
American Diabetes Association
October 28, 2008

"Economic Costs of Diabetes in the U.S. in 2007"
American Diabetes Association

Pancreas Image
Digestive Disorders Health Center
www.webmd.com/digestive-disorders/picture-of-the-pancreas

Diagnosis of Diabetes
National Institutes of Health
http://diabetes.niddk.nih.gov/dm/pubs/diagnosis

"Deaths among People with Diabetes, United States, 2006
National Institutes of Health
http://diabetes.niddk.nih.gov/dm/pubs/statistics

CHAPTER 2
"Diabetes – Disabling Disease to Double by 2050"
Source: Center for Disease Control
www.cdc.gov/needphp/publications/aag/ddt.htm

"Treating Diabetes"
National Diabetes Information Clearinghouse
www.diabetes.niddk.nih.gov

Treatment chart
2004-2006 National Health Interview Survey
National Institutes of Health
National Institute of Diabetes and Digestive and Kidney Diseases
http://diabetes.niddk.nih.gov/

"Failures of the US Health Care System
Life Extension
September 2008

"Consumer group asks government to ban Avandia"
American Diabetes Association
October 30, 2008

www.diabetes.org

"Diabetic Drug – FDA Puts Black Box Label on Rosiglitazone (Avandia)
Food & Drug Administration
Rockville, Maryland

"The Truth about Diabetes"
Walter Last
www.health-science-spirit.com/diabetestruth.htm

"Deaths Force NHlB1 to Drop Intensive Glucose-Lowering Strategy in Type 2 Diabetes"
Peggy Beck, Executive Editor
MedPage Today
February 6, 2008

"Diabetes Study Halted Due to Deaths"
ACCORD Study
National Institutes of Health

"Study: 2 diabetes drugs double fracture risk in women"
Steven Reinberg, HealthDay
The Detroit Free Press
December 10, 2008

"Tequin Diabetes Top Side Effect Leads to Defective Drug Lawsuit against
Bristol-Meyers
May 1, 2006
www.lawsuitsearch.com/drugs/tequin.aspx

Rezulin Side Effects – Lawsuits
www.rezulinnewsletter.com/html/effects.html

Diabetes treatment: Medications for Type 2 diabetes
January 26, 2009
Mayo Clinic
www.mayoclinic.com/health/diabetes-treatment

"Treating Diabetes"
National Institutes of Health
http://diabetes.niddk.nih.gov

"Medical care is 3rd leading cause of death in U.S.
JAMA: Journal of the American Medical Association
http://thehealthyskeptic.org
"Deaths among People with Diabetes, United States, 2006
CDC: Centers for Disease Control and Prevention

8th Annual HealthGrades Hospital Quality Study in America
HealthGrades
ScoutNews LLC
October 17, 2005

Report on Medication Errors
July 20, 2006
Institute of Medicine
The National Academies

"Diabetes Drugs: Summary of Recommendations"
Consumer Reports
www.consumerreports.org

Metformin
http://en.wikipedia.org/wiki/Metformin

Metformin Side Effects
http://diaetes.emedtv.com/metformin

BYETTA
ww.byetta.com

CHAPTER 3

"Treating Diabetes with Alternative Medicine"
http://diabetes.webmd.com

"Overeating Makes the Brain Go Haywire"
RedOrbit News

October 3, 2008
www.redorbit.com

"Alternative Treatments for Diabetes"
http://diabetes.webmd.com

"The Truth about Diabetes: The Sweet Connection"
www.health-science-spirit.com/diabetestruth.com

"Complementary and Alternative Medical Therapies for Diabetes"
National Center for Complementary and Alternative Medicine Clearinghouse
National Institute of Diabetes and Digestive and Kidney Diseases
http://diabetes.niddk.nih.gov/

"Natural Treatments for Type 2 Diabetes"
Cathy Wong
October 27, 2007
www.altmedicine.about.com/
"Traditional Chinese Medicine: Natural Remedies for Diabetes"
www.peacefulmind.com/diabetes.htm

Type 2 diabetes
www.mayoclinic.com

CHAPTER 7
"Healing with Low Level Laser Therapy" (January 2008)
Josephine Lee, MS, DC
The Health Planet

Nutritional Therapy 1:1 (2007)
www.nutritionaltherapycoop.com

Stratton IM, Adler Al, Neil HA, et al. Association of glycaemia with macro vascular and micro vascular complications of type 2 diabetes (UKPDS 35): prospective observational study. *BMJ*. 2000; 321:405-412.

Chapter 10

"Competence in wound healing, Diabetic Gangrene: Successful Therapy with RJ-Lasers"

www.rj-laser.com/english/diabetic.htm

ABOUT THE AUTHOR
DR. LARRY LYTLE

Raised on a South Dakota ranch during the Great Depression, Larry Lytle learned a basic understanding of the energy needed for healthy survival, as well as the common sense to understand the different components of health.

He graduated from Chadron State College in 1956 with a Bachelor of Science degree. He taught high school biology and coached basketball, after which he returned to college and received his DDS degree from the University of Nebraska in 1964. He then practiced dentistry in Rapid City, South Dakota until 1998.

During his dental career, Dr. Lytle earned Category II accredited status in the Academy of Laser Dentistry and was accredited in the American Academy of Cosmetic Dentistry. He also earned a PhD in nutrition in 1979 and provided nutritional consulting in conjunction with his dental practice. His general dental practice included cosmetic dentistry, laser dentistry, TMJ/TMD, and nutrition.

Dr. Lytle lectures and teaches in his many areas of expertise in the United States and abroad. In the area of proprioception, he was the developer of direct laser-bonded splints, Miracle Bite Tabs, and Easy Adjust Proprioceptive Guides. He also developed patents for low level lasers. He currently serves as a consultant for several companies in areas concerning proprioception to the brain and low level lasers, and conducts seminars around the world.

Dr. Lytle is a remarkably young and energetic man in his seventies. His combination of education, background, and real life experience help to ensure that you will read, re-read, and benefit from Universal Healer Book 2 Type II Diabetes for years to come.

Trained as an educator, he knows how to put complex information on many far-reaching topics and divergent health disciplines into one understandable whole.

As a practicing dentist for over thirty years and the sole remaining heir to the Dental Distress Syndrome legacy, created and initiated by the internationally renowned Al Fonder, DDS, Dr. Lytle incorporates little known factors regarding dental proprioception into his energy health system with amazing benefits for you.

After attaining his PhD in nutrition, Dr. Lytle incorporated whole body health into one of the most forward-thinking and acting preventive dental practices in the country.

Working, studying, writing, and teaching for the past decade in the alternative medical fields of energy medicine and low level laser therapy has put Dr. Lytle at the forefront of expertise in this area; his voice is one you should listen to in order to improve your health.

His main purpose in life has been to make a difference to mankind, and he passionately believes that *Universal Healer Book 2 Type II Diabetes* is an important tool for carrying out that goal.

It is health that is real wealth
And not pieces of gold and silver.

Mahatma Gandhi

Sometimes I get the feeling
the aspirin companies are
sponsoring my headaches.

V. L. Allineave